Praise for 7 Keys to

I love this book for many reasons. It's a book that helps you take action and enables you to learn about yourself. Taking check of where we are physically, emotionally, mentally and spiritually. This book is what people are searching for in their life, but are looking elsewhere, outside themselves! It's all right here, inside!

- Jill Shively, Author
Life Happens, Enjoy Your Journey!

If you need a quick and concise guide to your confusing and anxious feelings and emotions, this is it! This book is full of effective and easy-to-implement strategies to help you cope during these challenging times.

- Agnes Jackman, Founder,
OneLife Strategies

Dr. Elia Gourgouris - "The Happiness Doctor" and "Coach Kon" Apostolopoulos - authors of **7 Keys to Navigating a Crisis** *have done a wonderful job of utilizing their years of experience in counseling and coaching to share practical insights and tips for coping in a crisis. Not only will individuals and families find it useful, but also first responders, healthcare professionals, mental health counselors and wellness coaches as well. This book is an easy read and each chapter includes an end section with Points to Ponder, Questions to Consider, and Take Action ideas so the reader can go beyond just surviving to thriving, even in a crisis."*

- Randy McNeely, Author
The Kindness Givers' Formula

Dr. Elia and Coach Kon have given us a gift in the **7 Keys to Navigating a Crisis**. *Each chapter is filled with actionable steps to reframe our perspective and offer wisdom in times of chaos. A handy and useful tool I'll reach for time and again!*

- Lindy Rosenson, Owner ALR Speakers,
Private Manager to Elite Professional Speakers & Authors

7 Keys to Navigating a Crisis

A Practical Guide to Emotionally Dealing with Pandemics & Other Disasters

MAY YOUR JOURNEY BE FILLED
WITH GROWTH, FORGIVENESS AND MOST
OF ALL LOTS OF LOVE!!

Elia

Elia Gourgouris, PhD &
Konstantinos Apostolopoulos

7 Keys to Navigating a Crisis

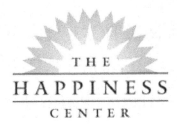

The Happiness Center
Superior, CO 80027

ISBN: 978-1-7349438-1-8

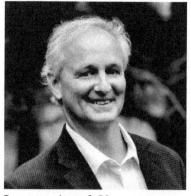

Dr. Elia Gourgouris is the Founder of **The Happiness Center** – an organization of world leading experts in the field of Positive Psychology dedicated to creating personal success and happiness.

Dr. Elia's previous book, **7 Paths to Lasting Happiness**, became an Amazon #1 best-seller. He is an International Keynote speaker and happiness expert focusing on corporate wellness & leadership training. He holds a PhD in Clinical Psychology and is a UCLA graduate. Dr. Elia is Certified by the American Red Cross in Disaster Mental Health Services having assisted in natural disasters and other crises, such as the 1994 Los Angeles and 2010 Haiti earthquakes, and the 1999 Columbine High School shooting. He's the co-host of The Kindness Happiness Connection and a Thrive Global contributor. He is spending the isolation period with his wife of 30 years, Sona and his young adult children in his home near Boulder, Colorado.

For more information:

Visit: **https://www.dreliagourgouris.com/**
Or **https://www.thehappinesscenter.com,**
LinkedIn: **https://www.linkedin.com/in/thehappinessdoctor/**

Konstantinos Apostolopoulos is the Founder & CEO of Fresh Biz Solutions, a performance consulting and training provider that helps businesses and institutions develop and manage their talent through tailored Human Capital Management strategies. Over the past 25 years, Coach Kon has been exploring and implementing best-practices to help organizations manage their transformational change efforts and prepare their leaders to handle difficult 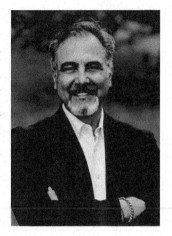 transitions. As an award-winning facilitator and coach, he has successfully delivered hundreds of custom learning events in the US, Canada, and Europe for diverse audiences and industries. He is a regular contributor to Thrive Global and other industry publications.

As a young man in Greece, he experienced firsthand the devastation left behind by natural and economic disasters. As an adult, he was fortunate to help play a small part in the rebuilding efforts in New Orleans after Hurricane Katrina. Today he helps others navigate the challenges brought by major events in their lives.

When not working with business leaders, Coach Kon gives back to his community by developing young soccer players in local, state, and Olympic Development Programs. Sports is a great way to teach life skills! During this extended isolation period, he is appreciating the time with his wife and daughter, while still looking for ways to make others smile.

For more information:

Email Coach Kon at: **kon@freshbizsolutions.com**
Visit: **www.freshbizsolutions.com**,
LinkedIn: **www.linkedin.com/in/coachkon**
or follow Coach Kon directly on Twitter (@Kon_Ap).

Dedication

To our families who help us navigate each crisis and give us a reason to persevere.

To all the people fighting to save lives, to those helping us all overcome the negative effects of the COVID-19 Pandemic, and to those just doing their part to put this crisis behind us.

Acknowledgements

We are deeply indebted to our families for their support, love, encouragement and sacrifice that allowed us to write this book during the COVID-19 Pandemic. It has been a labor of love that would not have been achievable without your constant reassurance that the time for this message is now, as humanity struggles to overcome from this unprecedented challenge.

A very special thank you to Randy McNeely for your invaluable assistance with navigating the twists and turns of the publishing process. Your professionalism and support are greatly appreciated.

Many thanks to Angie Alaya at pro_ebookcovers for the beautiful cover design. You are the consummate professional and a pleasure to work with.

Finally, we dedicate this book to all those individuals and families that have been affected deeply by the pandemic and those who will be affected by other natural disasters which will surely come. Traumatic events impact us personally and collectively as we are all part of the same race: the human race!

Elia Gourgouris PhD and Konstantinos Apostolopoulos
May 2020

Table of Contents

Introduction

Shortly after the beginning of 2020, the news reported a growing epidemic that was impacting a densely populated area of Wuhan Provence, China, at an alarming rate. It was identified as a new strain of the coronavirus, COVID-19. As the number of infected people grew, the disease quickly spread to other countries in the broader geographic area: South Korea, Singapore, Hong Kong, and Iran. Then it quickly surged to other parts of the world, including countries in Europe and the Americas, with Italy being hit overwhelmingly hard.

The numbers of those impacted – the sick, the dead, their communities and families – skyrocketed. The World Health Organization (WHO) quickly elevated this novel coronavirus to a Pandemic, as COVID-19 quickly spread to every continent, except for Antarctica. One after the other, local, State, and Federal governments declared a state of emergency. Measures to limit the spread of the virus became more desperate and people were expected to stay home and limit their movement. Was this a nightmare come true, or life imitating art?

The Flu Pandemic of 1918. Swine Flu. MERS. SARS. COVID-19 was the latest on a growing list of pandemics.

Hurricanes, cyclones, earthquakes, and tornadoes. Natural disasters with ever increasing ferocity and frequency that changed peoples' lives in an instant, not to mention global warming and the effects of pollution on the only planet we call home.

Wars, conflicts, horrific recurring acts of terrorism. Man-made disasters caused by people fighting one another for what they believed were just causes.

Financial scandals. Economic collapses. Recessions and depressions. The rapid cycling of the Bull and the Bear only compounded the ongoing world-wide anxiety.

The newswires now disburse stories of global disruptions that often either paralyze us with fear or just leave us feeling numb. It seems that the next crisis could be just around the corner, and we are left to deal with the emotional fall out. What can we do to better navigate these ongoing crises for ourselves, our families, our communities, our teams, and our organizations?

Compounding the problem

The growing crisis appears to exacerbate a less obvious, but still serious epidemic of mental health issues. According to Arianna Huffington's post, The Pandemic is Accelerating Our Mental Health Crisis, *"Even before anybody without a degree in epidemiology had ever heard of COVID-19, we were already in the middle of a mental health crisis. Worldwide, over **264 million people** were struggling with depression, and in the U.S. alone, nearly **50 million adults** had experienced some form of mental illness in the past year. And now, long periods of isolation, the loss of loved ones, the loss of jobs, financial insecurity and the daily stress of our new normal are accelerating that mental health crisis. Just as we've had to make drastic changes to our lives to stop the spread of the virus, we need to take urgent steps to safeguard our mental health, too."*

She further states these staggering statistics just one month into the Shelter-in-Place orders:

"To manage this new normal, many of us are reaching for short-term fixes that will only further damage our mental — and physical — health. As Sara Fischer writes in **Axios**, *Americans are 'doubling down on their worst habits to cope with the mental and emotional stress of the coronavirus pandemic.' Alcohol sales* **have jumped** *— with spirits up 75%, wine up 66% and beer up 42%. Cannabis use reached an* **all-time high** *in March — even as* **medical experts warn** *that marijuana and vaping, as well as tobacco, may increase the risk of COVID-19 infection and exacerbate the risks of spreading it. Not surprisingly, people are exercising less. They're also eating more and reaching for* **comfort foods** *— Oreos, Goldfish crackers, Slim Jims — with "COVID-15" becoming a meme for the standard quarantine weight gain.* **Scientists from Columbia University** *have warned that school closures could exacerbate already epidemic rates of childhood obesity, which in turn can have lifelong effects."*

Any light at the end of the tunnel now seems very small and distant. If this is the situation so early in the pandemic, what can we expect next? How can we navigate these uncharted waters more effectively than just escaping in unhealthy ways? There are things we can do to prepare emotionally, to deal with the challenges in a healthier way, and to minimize the negative effects of the crisis.

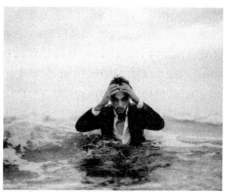

Image by Mubariz Mehdizadeh on Unsplash

Is it any wonder we feel this way?

It can help to visualize our capacity to handle stressful situations as a sponge, and those stressful situations as water pouring onto our "sponge." When we experience stress at a manageable rate, our sponge can absorb the water. But what if the water is flowing at a higher rate than what we can absorb? Then our sponge becomes saturated and struggles to absorb and contain the water. It becomes ineffective and can no longer handle the flowing water, rendering it, and us, incapacitated.

Much has been said and written about our "fight or flight" responses to perceived danger and stressful situations. Our system is wired to respond to these events and put us in a survival mode to protect us. Adrenaline floods our bloodstream, our breath quickens, and our body physically prepares to confront or run away from the threat. This has always been intended as a short-term response. But what happens when the short-term becomes the long-term, or even the new daily norm? Our adrenal glands become depleted and over-taxed. Our bodies struggle to recover and return to their neutral state. Our immune systems suffer; in essence, our "sponge" becomes saturated and ineffective.

When it comes to our mind and psyche, perception is reality. This means that our mind reacts to what it perceives is happening, whether that is real or not. Consider the rise of "virtual reality" as an effective tool for creating realistic simulations to train important skills, to provide an immersive experience, and solicit a specific emotional response. Our mind struggles to differentiate between what is real and not and reacts accordingly. We watch an image of someone on a high building, and as the camera follows him or her approach the edge of the balcony, that tingling feeling low in our stomach starts to grow. The lens peers over the edge and we go weak at the knees! Our mind is responding to the image, to the perception, even though we are nowhere near that edge.

This example illustrates the power of perception. Therefore, how we view a particular situation will determine how we respond to it. Do we perceive a threat, danger, or a stressful situation? Then we will respond accordingly. Do we feel in control or at ease? Then we will respond according to that perception. Again, our perception will determine our response. Not just our perception of the environment and circumstances, but also our perception of how well we believe we can cope with the environment and circumstances. Have we successfully dealt with this situation before? Have we failed to handle this challenge in the past? Is the glass half-full, or half-empty? The answers to these questions will impact how we approach the current situation or challenge.

> *Your own resolution to success is more important than any other thing.*
>
> *- Abraham Lincoln*

The good news is that we have a choice. We can choose how we respond to each <u>new</u> challenge. With each experience we have the power to learn and grow, to overcome past failures, and to gain confidence in our ability to handle adversity. That is part of our evolutionary human nature.

However, the questions remain. Are there helpful ways to navigate these ongoing crises for ourselves, our families, our communities, our teams, and our organizations? If so, what are they?

The answer, of course, is yes there are helpful ways to navigate this crisis. In this book we provide seven powerful keys to navigating the current pandemic as well as natural disasters, and other global disruptions.

Why are we writing this book?

Anytime there is a crisis, we all have the opportunity to help others using our unique talents and gifts. It can be as simple as a smile or a kind word, an offer to help carry goods to those in need, or even the sacrifice of those on the front line – soldiers, firefighters, police officers, or medical staff. But also, those that simply keep things going for the rest of us by stocking shelves at the stores, delivering food and medicines, producing life's necessities, and keeping the lights on.

In the past we have both been in situations that have called for a committed pair of hands to assist, a willing ear to listen, and even a friendly shoulder to cry on. We have experienced personal loss in our lives, and we understand the emotions that come with great upheaval and tragedy. We have each battled our own demons and have helped others to overcome challenges in their lives. We have been athletes and worked with athletes to help them achieve their best. Collectively we have more than 60 years of hands-on experience teaching and coaching, of working with individuals and teams, to help them achieve their goals and do our part to make things better.

At this time, in April 2020 and at the height of the growing COVID-19 Pandemic in the US, we felt compelled to share our thoughts and experiences in the hope that others might benefit and that it might help them navigate this and future crises. We also share the roles that many others play as parents, spouses, siblings, leaders, business owners, and neighbors. We understand that there are so many emotions and questions going through our minds in this turbulent time. There are so many sources of information out there – many helpful, some less so. We hope to provide you with a simple read with practical tips, to help you get through these times, and to even go beyond surviving to truly thriving. We hope that you will find insight, compassion, and even a few smiles in the words and stories included in this book. We hope that you realize you are not alone, and that we're here to help.

How is this book different?

Most self-help books have wonderful ideas and inspiring concepts. But what usually happens after we read a book like that? If we only read it, highlight a few things, and put it away on a shelf when we're finished, then very little will change. If that's the kind of book you're looking for, this isn't it. We know many people who are knowledgeable and highly educated, yet who are quite unprepared in their lives.

They know intellectually the steps to emergency preparedness, but knowledge without application is just education. I can read the top 10 books on how to prepare for a crisis, and underline and highlight them to death. If I don't act upon what they say, I'll still be in the same position I was in before I read them, just more knowledgeable and probably a lot more frustrated with my circumstances. You can learn all the things that contribute to being prepared like self-care, flexibility, staying positive, and being kind in the midst of a crisis, but if you don't apply them in your life, not much will change.

This book was written specifically as a practical guide with reader engagement in mind. For that purpose, at the end of each chapter you will find specific points to ponder, questions to consider and answer, and calls to action. We can assure you that as you earnestly implement these actions, your capacity to navigate the current crisis, as well as future crises, will greatly increase.

Let's get started!

Before diving into the rest of the book, we invite you to take the following assessment to help you evaluate your starting point. It will give you an indication of your *current*, personal health in four important areas of well-being:

- Physical

- Mental

- Emotional

- Spiritual

The most important part of this process is to be honest and fair when answering each question. Remember that this will give you your entry point, not your final result. As with life, it's not how you start, it's how you finish. And we are here to help you navigate these turbulent times and finish strong!

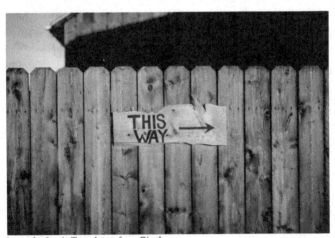

Image by Jamie Templeton from Pixabay

Personal Health Assessment[1]

Physical Health   1 poor – 5 excellent

How is your energy throughout the day?   1 2 3 4 5

How rested do you feel when you wake   1 2 3 4 5
up in the morning?

How healthy is your diet?   1 2 3 4 5

How is your level of daily activity and 1 2 3 4 5
exercise?

How well do you function without   1 2 3 4 5
escaping?
   (I don't use alcohol, drugs, smoking,
caffeine, when stressed)

Mental Health

How is your ability to maintain a   1 2 3 4 5
positive attitude?

How is your ability to stay focused right 1 2 3 4 5
now?

How good are you at keeping life's   1 2 3 4 5
events in perspective?

How grateful do you feel right now?   1 2 3 4 5

How open are you to hearing other   1 2 3 4 5
people's insights/opinions?
   (Especially when they are different
from yours)

---

[1] © Copyright 2020, Elia Gourgouris, Ph.D.

Emotional Health

How well do you practice self-compassion / self-forgiveness?	1	2	3	4	5
How well do you maintain a healthy life-work balance?	1	2	3	4	5
How well can you maintain flexibility under stress?	1	2	3	4	5
How much is humor, laughter, and playfulness part of your daily life?	1	2	3	4	5
How healthy are your relationships?	1	2	3	4	5

Spiritual Health

How strong is your belief in a positive outcome?	1	2	3	4	5
How close do you feel to God or your higher power?	1	2	3	4	5
How much do you pray, meditate or practice mindfulness?	1	2	3	4	5
How often do you practice kindness or do acts of service towards others?	1	2	3	4	5
How well do you know and live your purpose in life?	1	2	3	4	5

Please add all your answers to calculate your score: Total Score =

Interpreting your score:

There are two ways to interpret your score. The first is your cumulative score, which gives you an indication of your overall sense of health, fulfillment, and happiness in life:

- 81-100: I am generally healthy and happy in my life. Feedback in specific areas might be useful.

- 65-80: My life is okay, but not always what I would like it to be. I could use some direction in making my life healthier.

- 50-65: My life is not going in a direction I would like it to go. I need guidance in learning how to have greater health and wellness.

- Less than 50: My life is unhealthy and needs to change now. (Don't give up – this is a great opportunity for growth!)

The second way to interpret your score has to do with the individual areas which are covered in the survey. Research has shown that the twenty areas addressed in the questions are specific indicators which contribute to one's overall sense of wellness. So, for example, if a score was less than 4 on a particular question, it shows room for improvement in that specific area. The lower the score, the greater the opportunity for growth.

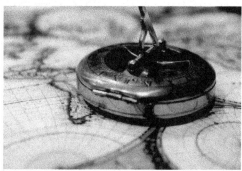

Image by schaeffter from Pixabay

Points to Ponder:

- I can control my thoughts
- I can control my attitude
- I can control the way I view life.

Questions to Consider:

What am I willing to do today, to be better prepared?

- If I start right now, where will I be in a week or a month or a year, as opposed to just letting the status quo continue?

Take Action:

- Make a conscious decision that you have a choice.
- Determine what aspects of the current crisis are within your control and what are not. Take a sheet of paper and divide the page into two columns.
  - In column A write down all the things you feel are beyond your control. For example, a) the pandemic b) Federal, state and local restrictions of movement, c) kids being at home instead of school, d) being laid off and so on.
  - In column B write down all the things that are within your control. For example, a) Your attitude towards these events (which then leads to a lot more options that are within your control), b) enjoying the time with your family, c) going for walks, d) connecting with loved ones via social media and so on.
- Put a plan in place on how to best prepare and organize your day. (You can update your plan once you read *Key #5 Preparation*)

Key #1: Self-Care

Self-care is a critical element when navigating a crisis. Anyone that has travelled on an airplane has heard the flight attendant's safety announcement before take-off. Regardless of the airline, one of the things that remains constant is the direction *"to put on our own oxygen mask first before helping others"*. Why is that? Because we can't help others if we are struggling to breath, unconscious, or otherwise incapacitated! We can't help others if we're not OK.

There are many things we can do to care for ourselves and preserve our health. Take for example the recent announcement from the World Health Organization regarding the basic tips to keep ourselves safe and help contain the spread of the virus.

☐ Wash your hands with soap and water for 20 seconds.

☐ Avoid touching your face, eyes, mouth, and nose.

☐ Avoid contact with people who are vulnerable. And if you can, wear a mask.

☐ Cover your cough with the bend of your elbow.

☐ Disinfect surfaces you regularly use.

☐ If you feel unwell, stay at home and call your healthcare provider.

☐ Only share information from trusted sources.

How well are you following these guidelines? Are you protecting yourself and those around you? Place a checkmark by the recommended safety tips you want to focus on and make a habit.

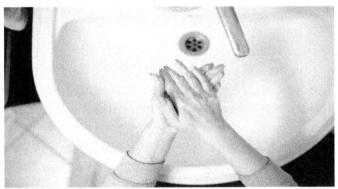

Image by Martin Slavoljubovsky from Pixabay

Care for Your (Inner) Child

Basically, **mismanagement of stress is a long-term neglect of our needs**. Long-term exposure to stress can make us physically sick or lead to emotional and mental breakdowns. How do we change our mindset from being overwhelmed by dealing with a crisis to taking charge of our lives? We need to stop, reflect and meditate on the direction of our work, our

family, and every other aspect of our lives. It's a key ingredient to successfully managing our overall stress levels.

Setting limits on ourselves can help to eliminate some of the stressors in our lives. For example, if you're struggling with overcommitment, part of learning to set limits is having the ability to say "no" and not feeling guilty about it. (Dr. Elia): *When I was younger, I didn't have the ability to say "no" because I was a people-pleaser. As I have gotten older, saying "no" has become a lot easier for me. Given the increased demands on my time, I've learned to say "no" as a way of taking care of myself.* If you fall in the people-pleasing category, every time you say *"No"* to someone/something, you're saying *"Yes"* to your self-care.

Over-commitment increases our stress levels, and our relationships, our health and our productivity will suffer. We then feel overwhelmed, and our stress level increases even more. Setting limits on our activities is a part of self-preservation. It's so easy to run ourselves ragged! Much like a racecar, we can't operate at full speed indefinitely, because we'll blow a gasket. Either something will crack physically, or we'll be mentally or emotionally drained. A nervous breakdown could be around the corner. That is the inevitable result from long-term exposure to a high amount of stress.

Interestingly, with the COVID-19 pandemic we are facing a different set of circumstances that are unprecedented in peacetime. Having our movement restricted by the local, State, and Federal government(s), hunkering down, unable to go to work presents a different set of stressors. In this case we might find ourselves with *too much time* on our hands and not enough to do. We might feel unproductive, empty, or even depressed – especially as the economic impact of these restrictions begins to take its toll on us and our families. As we become inundated by the continuous flow of (mostly negative) information, **the stress surrounding our physical wellbeing is compounded by the anxiety created for our financial wellbeing!**

What we really need to do is **parent ourselves**. Most parents don't neglect their kids – they're very mindful of their needs, especially when they're young. They feed them, clothe them, bathe them, love them, and get them to bed at a reasonable hour. But how many of us are good at parenting ourselves? When working with clients who are neglecting themselves, we've found it's very effective to compare the way they treat themselves to the way they take care of their children. For example, if a person is so busy that they forget to eat, we'll ask them, "*Can you imagine not feeding your child breakfast and lunch tomorrow?*" Of course, they're always shocked at the prospect, but then we point out that that's what they're doing to themselves! If we ask them why they take care of their children, the response is always, "*I have to! If I don't, then who will?*" We then point out that the same principle applies to us as adults: if we don't take care of ourselves, who will? Sometimes we're so busy we deprive ourselves of the most fundamental things: sleep and food. Can you imagine having the following conversation with your child?

> You: *You need to be on your phone until 2:00 a.m. and keep checking your social media!*

> Your Child: *But Mom/Dad, I'm tired, I want to go to sleep!*

> You: *NO! Keep checking your phone to see if you got any more likes!* LOL

How often do we say to ourselves, "*Go to bed! You need your sleep?*" We frequently say it to our children; to ourselves, not nearly enough. And even more importantly, we need to listen and follow through, so plug that phone in (away from your bed) and leave it there!

Setting limits and parenting ourselves is the ultimate expression of self-compassion and self-care.

From NIMBI to IMBI

When a decision between a short-term temptation is at odds with our long-term welfare, do we choose long-term welfare? This principle is typically known as self-discipline, viewed through the consciousness of wanting to build a better future, one decision at a time. We like to call it the "**NIMBI Principle**" (Not In My Best Interest!) Any time we give in to self-destructive behavior, we are hurting ourselves. Since we all have areas where we need to improve, how can we best make use of this wonderful little phrase? When might this be applicable in your life? Siblings, spouses, relatives, or other well-meaning people in our lives may sometimes offer enticements. For example, if you've been trying to quit smoking, a friend might offer you a cigarette, possibly not knowing you've committed to stop.

From now on, whenever somebody asks you to do something you know deep down inside isn't in your best interest, remember the NIMBI Principle, and turn down the invitation. What I love about this simple saying is how empowering it feels to say it. Could you say it without judgment, but with a smile?

"It's midnight, more cake anyone?" *"**NIMBI!**"*

"Want to smoke?" *"**NIMBI!**"*

"Want to stay up all night with worry and stress about the pandemic?" Again, *"**NIMBI!**"*

By choosing what's right for ourselves, we're taking care of ourselves. And that's an important part of loving ourselves. I hope we can make this part of our daily lexicon. It will bless our lives and maybe even give others permission to do the same. *"**NIMBI: It's not in my best interest!**"* What a lovely phrase!

So now let's transition from **NIMBI** to **IMBI** (In My Best Interest). Think about what <u>is</u> in your best interest during a crisis. Perhaps if we're limited to our homes without much to do, we could give ourselves permission to take a nap. Multiple studies support the benefits of taking a daily nap. It reduces stress, refreshes not only our bodies but our minds as well. This simple act can make such a difference in our mood, our physical energy, and mental clarity, while reinforcing the idea of self-care! Or how about taking more time to connect with family members and friends through phone calls, texts, or emails? Take a walk, read that book you've been putting off, watch that documentary, play some games with fellow housemates, maybe even have your own in-home film festival!

Self-Care for Healthcare

Every year especially in the summertime there are catastrophic wildfires consuming millions of acres of land across the world. On the frontlines, firefighters battle tirelessly to protect our homes, business and our very lives, often putting their own lives at risk. Now the world is facing a different wildfire, unlike anything we've seen in recent human history. The Coronavirus pandemic has spread to virtually every corner of the earth. Nobody seems to have escaped this unseen threat to our very lives. The consequences of this new form of wildfire have been devastating.

On the front lines our modern-day super-heroes, doctors, nurses and other health care practitioners are giving it their all to protect us and our communities. Oftentimes with limited resources, such as lack of protective gear, masks, gowns and the all too critical ventilators. Doctors are facing the horrific dilemma of who lives and who dies in certain of the hardest hit areas around the world. They often do it at the peril of their own health and unfortunately even their very lives. Tens of thousands of health care practitioners have been infected by this virus.

As coronavirus cases jump and deaths surge in Italy, new figures show an "enormous" level of contagion among the country's medical personnel. Thousands of health workers have been infected by coronavirus since the onset of the outbreak, representing 8.3 percent of total cases. The data has sent shock waves through the country's already strained healthcare system. According to Director Nino Cartabellotta, a public health expert:

"We already have a limited number of doctors and nurses. Under extreme circumstances, we could even ask them to keep working even if [they] tested positive for coronavirus. Still, they should be equipped with protective devices to avoid spreading the virus further. We are importing medical personnel from abroad and throwing new young healthcare professionals without licenses into the fray. If we don't provide them with adequate protection, it will end up like in a war where soldiers don't die while fighting on the battlefield, but because of lack of equipment. The more medical personnel are infected, the weaker the responsiveness of the healthcare system."

Healthcare professionals are literally working around the clock, sometimes up to 36 hours straight before they either collapse or physically cannot stay awake. There are several reports of doctors and nurses who died in China, not because of the virus but because of pure exhaustion! Of course, these are extreme examples and hopefully isolated cases. But what can nurses and doctors do in order to protect themselves, not just physically but emotionally and mentally, while they are on the front lines fighting this pandemic?

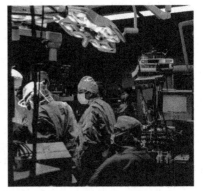

Image by Piron Guillaume from Unsplash

In an effort to support our front-line heroes, doctors, nurses, and other health practitioners to stay physically healthy, mentally strong, emotionally centered, and spiritually grounded, we propose a **Self-care for Healthcare guide**: practical ways to strengthen healthcare professionals' abilities to perform their duties at peak performance during these tremendously challenging times.

The following tips for the mental, emotional, spiritual and physical areas are found in Dr. Terry Lyles' *Stress Recovery – A disaster Relief Manual*. Dr Lyles and I (Dr. Elia), are both colleagues and friends; we had the opportunity to work together to help provide humanitarian assistance to the people of Haiti after their devastating earthquake in 2010. Since I have been certified through the American Red Cross for Disaster Relief Emotional Preparedness, I assisted Dr. Lyles at an orphanage and helped those on the front lines with the following plan that focuses on the whole person, by addressing four important areas of well-being:

1. **Physical**

    a. Take regular breaks every 90 minutes, even if it's just for a few minutes.

    b. Drink water regularly; it is critical to stay well hydrated and balanced.

    c. Eat small but frequent meals or snacks of healthy, low-fat, low-sugar foods, with little food prior to bedtime. Food has a direct impact on our mood. Healthy food will help calm nerves and tension, whereas junk food can agitate and create negative mood such as depression and anxiety.

    d. Do some stretching exercises and breathing to help keep you grounded and focused.

e. Do your best to go to bed at the same time each night. Prior to falling asleep focus on positive thoughts and expect a restful and restorative sleep experience.

2. **Mental**

   a. Focus on what is in your control, not what is out of your control.

   b. Look for the positive in every situation.

   c. See how much you are helping and know that you and your colleagues are doing the absolute best that you can at this time.

   d. Before going to sleep think about, or write down, all the victories you witnessed or were part of during the day. Remember that small things add up over time; keeping track will help you stay focused on the positives.

   e. Certain conditions are truly temporary so see them as such.

3. **Emotional**

   a. Talk to someone about how you are feeling. If you need support in any area: mental, emotional, spiritual or physical, ask for help or have someone just listen. Make a list of people you feel comfortable talking with.

   b. Allow yourself to feel your feeling. Pushing them down will only cover them up and could result in sickness.

   c. Write letters or keep a journal to help process the trauma of your experience.

   d. Make a list of what you are grateful for and add to it each day. When you are feeling low, refer to the list.

4. **Spiritual**

   a. Focus on your purpose as a health care practitioner and on your purpose in life; it will give you the inspiration to continue.

b. Remember the "big picture" while handling the little details of the day.

c. See yourself as a humanitarian who was sent to help those in need.

d. Ask yourself why you are alive, and then discover how to help someone else in need.

e. Have faith and trust that good things will come out of this disaster.

f. Take time to talk to God or your Higher Power and ask for spiritual guidance, then share how you feel.

We strongly believe that this guide is not only applicable for healthcare professionals, but all of us dealing with challenges on the front lines of our lives and those of our loved ones.

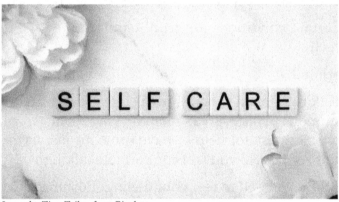

Image by Tiny Tribes from Pixabay

Points to Ponder:

- I will follow the safety guidelines for myself, my loved ones, and those around me.

- I will take care of myself and my needs, so that I can help others in turn.

- I will consider how to incorporate the NIMBI Principle in my life.

Questions to Consider:

- What emotional responses am I feeling during this time of crisis? Am I experiencing grief?

- What about those around me? Are they experiencing grief?

- How well do I nurture and "parent" myself?

Take Action:

- Follow the guidelines of the WHO with exactness! (This is not the time to pick and choose. Unfortunately, we do not have that luxury).

- Set healthy limits and boundaries to avoid draining my physical, mental, and emotional energy. How can I say NO when necessary, without feeling guilty? (Remember that when you say NO to unreasonable expectations, you're saying YES to yourself).

- Be kind and loving to myself, as a good parent to a child.

Key #2: Awareness

When we look for answers to our most pressing questions, we seek council from those we trust the most – perhaps a parent, a sibling, a friend, a mentor, a confidante, a teacher, or a coach. How many times do we stop and listen to our intuition, our inner voice, our spirit, to help us solve our everyday problems and seek answers that set the direction for our lives? So often, our intuition can just cut through all the static and speak to us from the very core of our being and reveal the truth that we would have never experienced if we hadn't been paying attention.

How do we find those answers that are in alignment with our beliefs and our values? Those answers don't usually leap up to greet us when we are moving at a million miles an hour! The first thing we need to do is slow down, quiet our mind, and open up, to really experience and then understand what's happening around us and inside us. It's amazing what you hear and understand when you slow down enough to really see and listen.

There is a voice that doesn't use words.
Listen!

— Rumi, 13th century Persian poet

It's of no use to move ahead, until you have a good idea where you're going. It's a poor use of your time, to solve the wrong problem or find an answer to the wrong question. The answer to the right questions simply won't come to us if we're not listening. So quiet down your mind, open up your heart, and listen to your inner truth. From our personal experience, we can tell you that EVERY time we have listened to that voice and then acted; it has ALWAYS worked out. We wish we could honestly say that we have always listened but being imperfect human beings, there have been times in our lives when we disregarded the *"voice"*. Guess what outcome we received? The wrong one! And we paid dearly for it. Hopefully as we get older and gain more experience, we will make an even greater effort to get quiet, listen to that voice, and act upon its wisdom. It won't let you down, we promise you that!

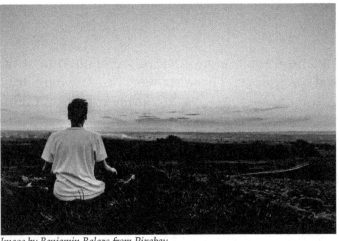

Image by Benjamin Balazs from Pixabay

In the same way, we can't take care of ourselves if we don't recognize what might be wrong. If we remain aware of our physical and emotional condition, we can quickly identify areas that might require attention and care. Then we can act to regain our balance and well-being.

What is a potentially traumatic event?

Potentially traumatic events can be caused by a singular occasion, or from ongoing, relentless stresses. A potentially traumatic event is more prone to leave an individual with longer-lasting emotional and psychological trauma if:

- The individual was unprepared for the event
- The event itself was completely unexpected
- The person felt powerless to prevent the event

While traumatic experiences frequently involve life-threatening events, any situation that leaves one feeling alone and completely overwhelmed can be traumatic – even without physical harm. It's important to remember that it's not the objective facts of the event alone that determine how traumatic an event is; it's also the subjective emotional experience of the event. Often, the more terror and helplessness one feels, the more likely it is that an individual will be traumatized.

Signs and Symptoms of Emotional and Psychological Trauma

Potentially traumatic events are defined as events that are both powerful and upsetting that intrude into one's daily life. They can involve a major threat to one's psychological and physical well-being and may be life-threatening to one's own life or the life of a loved one. These events may have very little impact on one individual but can lead to significant distress in another.

Examples of events and situations that can lead to the development of psychological trauma may include:

- Natural disasters such as fires, earthquakes, tornados, and hurricanes

- Pandemics like COVID-19

- Financial ruin or distress due to sudden unemployment

Many people experience strong physical or emotional reactions immediately following the experience of a traumatic event, but most will notice that their feelings dissipate over the course of a few days or weeks. However, for some individuals, the symptoms of psychological trauma may be increasingly severe and last longer. This may be the result of the nature of the traumatic event, availability of emotional support, past and present life stressors, personality types, and available coping mechanisms. Some of the most common symptoms of psychological trauma may include the following:

Cognitive:

- Intrusive thoughts of the event that may occur out of the blue
- Nightmares
- Visual images of the event
- Loss of memory and concentration abilities
- Disorientation
- Confusion
- Mood swings

Behavioral:

- Avoidance of activities or places that trigger memories of the event
- Social isolation and withdrawal
- Lack of interest in previously enjoyable activities

Physical:

- Easily startled
- Tremendous fatigue and exhaustion
- Tachycardia
- Edginess
- Insomnia
- Chronic muscle patterns
- Sexual dysfunction
- Changes in sleeping and eating patterns
- Vague complaints of aches and pains throughout the body
- Extreme alertness; always on the lookout for warnings of potential danger

Psychological:

- Overwhelming fear
- Obsessive and compulsive behaviors
- Detachment from other people and emotions
- Emotional numbing
- Depression
- Guilt – especially if one lived while others perished
- Shame
- Emotional shock
- Disbelief
- Irritability
- Anger
- Anxiety
- Panic attacks

These symptoms can take days, weeks, or even months to develop, and it's not uncommon for us to experience more than one of them at any given point. That's why self-awareness (our ability to look inside and assess) is so important in recognizing these behaviors and initiating our response. In other words, we might be ok with being told to self-isolate for a few days. But when days become weeks – or even months! – then many of the symptoms listed above will most likely become commonplace and magnified.

Acknowledge your own reactions

It's difficult to move forward in a crisis unless we understand our thoughts and feelings about it – both positive and negative. If we ignore our initial reactions, they may surface later, paralyzing us and preventing us from taking any action at all.

We can start by identifying and describing our thoughts and feelings. This is a process of self-examination that we can do on our own or with a trusted partner, someone with whom we feel comfortable and who can help us think through our reactions.

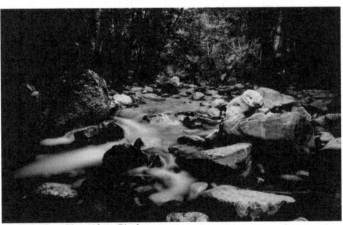

Image by Free-Photos from Pixabay

Transitions and Stages of Grief

Part of caring for ourselves and others in a time of crisis, is understanding and working through the personal and human side of change. Our lives are being changed and impacted by so many things: fear, distancing, isolation, shortage of goods on the shelves, loss of income, people getting sick and dying.

In his book *Managing Transitions*, William Bridges explains that change, like so many other things in life, has a beginning, a middle, and an ending. When it comes to life's changes though, the expected order of things is reversed. First, we experience the **Ending** of what currently is, a deep sense of loss and grief. Then we experience the **Neutral Zone**, the feeling of uncertainty and being up in the air while nothing seems concrete anymore. And finally, we experience the **New Beginning**, when we finally accept the new reality and circumstances.

We cannot underestimate the feelings that come with a major change or crisis. The bigger and more unexpected the change, the deeper the grief. In a time of crisis, like a global pandemic, the feelings can be multiplied as the changes and the **stages of grief** are experienced by many at the same time. We can clearly recognize these stages in ourselves and others:

- **Stage 1** – Disbelief and Denial: Typically, the first reaction is extreme shock. We may deny that things will change, despite news and announcements. Even when the effects of the crisis are being experienced by those around us, we may strive to convince ourselves that nothing will change. Not for us. As an example, initially the Covid-19 virus was limited to China and then parts of Asia. Even then most people in the US and Europe felt like "surely this isn't going to affect us too."

- **Stage 2** – Anger Through Rage and Resentment. As reality of the situation becomes more obvious, feelings of shock and disbelief are replaced by anger and resentment toward those considered responsible. We may direct our anger towards an individual, a certain group of people, the disease, the government, or even the world in general. We look to place blame and criticize "others", whomever those others may be.

- **Stage 3** – Emotional Bargaining, Beginning in Anger and Ending in Depression. As uncertainty drives fear about our future, anger often turns inward. We can become angry with ourselves for not seeing the crisis coming or anticipating the fallout of the events. We may come to resent our own behavior for not "fighting" harder for our rights, or even feel victimized by others and the situation. Often, we become nostalgic for what is past or what 'used to be'. Feelings of anger may subside to be replaced with depression. For example, "what about my sports, missing graduation, or my summer vacation?" "I have already made plans to go visit family and friends". "I was so looking forward to that, why did this happen to me/us?"

- **Stage 4** – Acceptance. Finally, we recognize that what is past may be gone forever and begin to accept the new reality. This doesn't mean we agree, but rather they we are willing to accept what is being said or done. Specifically, the restriction of movement, quarantines, social distancing, remote work environment and rationing of supplies (think about the mad dash to secure toilet paper and hand sanitizer). Psychologically acceptance is the healthier stage for us to reach. Once we accept the new realities on the ground, we can begin to more rationally prepare to deal with the current crisis.

Faith vs. Fear

All human emotions find their genesis in either the "**Faith Camp**," or the "**Fear Camp**." Stress, anxieties, depression, pessimism, discouragement, anger, loneliness and mistrust are all members of the fear camp. A recent national survey found that 75 percent of Americans are stressed, anxious and angry. Those numbers have likely skyrocketed during the time of the Coronavirus Pandemic. Undoubtedly, every one of us has "visited" the Fear Camp at least occasionally in our lifetime. The point is not that we shouldn't be fearful or that we shouldn't set foot in the fear camp. It is part of the human experience and is entirely normal. The point is that we shouldn't remain there permanently. In fact, it really should be one of our goals to make fewer and shorter "visits" to the Fear Camp.

> *When you are going through something hard and wonder where God is, remember the teacher is always quiet during a test.*
>
> *– Unknown*

If, for example, a person is generally feeling stressed for months at a time, maybe they can reduce it to a few weeks. If feelings of inadequacy ruled their life for weeks at a time, how much would their life improve if that could be reduced to just a few days? Instead of feeling discouraged for days on end, try wallowing in the muck for just one day. How do we get out of the fear camp? The answer is most importantly, to become aware of our negative thoughts. Once we can begin to recognize them as they come up, we need to choose to limit them (I will allow myself a "pity party" for one hour today, before I need to move on). And lastly, begin to move on by taking action.

<u>Choose</u> to believe in a positive outcome by visiting the "**Faith Camp**" – by having faith.

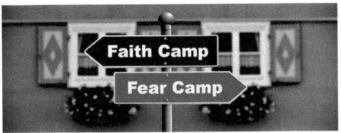

Original Image by Gerd Altmann from Pixabay

Some of the attributes found in the Faith Camp include hope, optimism, security, confidence, trust, happiness and peace. When visiting the Faith Camp, we are comforted. Faith is remaining at peace, **even** while in the middle of the storm. When everything seems to go wrong; when our dreams, aspirations, expectations or plans go awry, what will we choose to believe - fear? Or will we consciously choose to have faith that things will turn out all right? This can happen as we begin to watch and train our thoughts, and then re-direct and replace the negative and fearful ones into positive and faith-filled thoughts. Allow your "adult" side to comfort and over-ride the more fearful "child" in you. The happy person chooses faith over fear and enjoys wonderful benefits of doing so.

Worrying is actually having a lack of faith. Our lives don't need to be left to chance. We do have a choice to make and choosing faith will have the greatest positive impact on how we live. Even though it's difficult, choosing faith can immediately eliminate the fear. If we want to go from just surviving to thriving, faith is the only way! How do we visit the "Faith Camp?" Sometimes we can't get there by ourselves, no matter how hard we try. It may take active prayer and meditation – appealing to God or our higher power – to restore the sense of peace in our heart that everything is going to be okay and that everything will turn out all right.

There has never been a time in recent human history when our faith collectively has been tested as it is during this pandemic. Thousands of people are dying or getting sick every single day all over the world. If ever there was an opportunity for us to choose faith over fear, now is the time! So, let us choose faith which brings us inner peace and reduces our worry and stress.

Faith is taking the first step even when you can't see the whole staircase.

— Dr. Martin Luther King, Jr.

Points to Ponder:

- Be aware of your emotional and physical reactions during stressful times.

- Be aware that only danger is real; fear is an emotional response that can paralyze us.

- Be aware of the choice: Fear Camp or Faith Camp. Which will you visit?

Questions to Consider:

- What is your inner voice telling you?

- What would you do if you weren't afraid?

- What would you tell a child to comfort them, and can you give that same advice to your own inner child?

Take Action:

- Whether we are working on our own or with a partner, a good way to get our feelings out is to put them on paper. We can describe the challenge or crisis at the top of a piece of paper and divide the page into two columns labeled "pros" and "cons".

- In the positive column, list every potential positive outcome you can think of. In the other column, list your fears and concerns.

- Place a check mark next to the things you can control or do something about.

- Commit to taking action that will help you realize one positive or minimize one negative from the things check marked.

What's the challenge or crisis I'm facing?	
Pros	Cons
•	•

Key #3: Flexibility

Improvise, adapt, and overcome. This is a popular mantra in the US Armed Forces that resonates with the times we are experiencing now. In many ways it feels like a war against an enemy that we can't see, we can't hear, and we can't even identify until we are hit. The best way to overcome the effects of the virus seems to be, (if possible) to not get it. All the authorities are telling us to simply stay away from the infection. To minimize our exposure, and shelter in place. To isolate. To quarantine.

Most of us have come to expect a few limits on our freedom. We have fought wars to earn that right, yet now we are asked to relinquish it and self-isolate. This has created a sense of resentment in many that can be directed inward or outward, as we shift blame from ourselves to others. We engage in emotional responses that offer few solutions but remain a normal part of being human. To allow us to move forward, it's important to acknowledge these reactions and understand why we're experiencing them. With the understanding of why we feel a certain way, we can process the emotions and act to move ourselves into a better place.

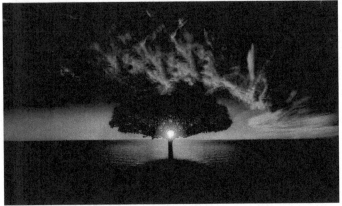

Image by Bessi from Pixabay

Four Responses to Unexpected or Rapid Change

When we experience the kind of rapid change that occurs in a crisis, it can elevate our stress levels significantly. Our own response to this forced change may vary from situation to situation. Consider the following four typical responses[2] that are all normal and legitimate.

Victim Mode

When we are in the *Victim Mode*, we find ourselves feeling angry or depressed, isolating and failing to ask for help, fighting and resisting change to our routines. We are flooded by emotions and we ask: *Why is this happening to me again? Why can't things stay the way they are?* The victim mode is the most disempowering one because it's plagued by feelings of *"I don't have much of a choice"* and *"poor me."*

Critic Mode

---

[2] Although many studies have been conducted on how people respond to change, there is no single, agreed-upon model. The Four Responses to Change described here are based on Peter Block's Stewardship: Choosing Service over Self-Interest (San Francisco, Barrett-Koehler Publishers, Inc., 1993), pp. 221-231

When we are in the *Critic Mode,* we are looking for reasons why the efforts to make things better will not be successful. We fail to see any positive outcomes from the situation, while we also question and challenge whether any change is appropriate or necessary. We may find ourselves saying, *"This hasn't worked so far, and I don't think it will work now",* or *"I doubt what they're proposing will improve anything."* Playing the blame-game has never been an effective way to manage stress, and it expands the already negative rhetoric. Choose to be part of the solution, not part of the problem!

Bystander Mode

When we are in the *Bystander Mode,* we feel reluctant to get involved, waiting for others to make decisions and take the lead. We think to ourselves, *"If I ignore this crisis, it will go away",* and we bury our head in the sand and remain in denial. Other times we wait until we see how this impacts other people first, or we simply refuse to act until we don't have a choice. Unfortunately, this refusal to actively participate and be part of the solution can be detrimental to our physical, emotional, and mental health.

Navigator Mode

When we are in the *Navigator Mode,* we look for ways to minimize the negative effects of the crisis on ourselves and others. As we explore the underlying issues, we also look for opportunities to make things better, find ways to be useful and supportive to others, and form nurturing relationships with others affected by the crisis. So, the goal is for all of us to shift from these different modes until we can get to the *Navigator Mode*: the one which can take us from just surviving to thriving!

It is common for our response to shift during a crisis. We could be in the *Navigator Mode* when a crisis first hits but revert to the *Victim Mode* as we personally experience more of the effects of the crisis. What's most important is not to get stuck in the

Victim, Critic, or *Bystander Mode* – all of which inhibit forward movement.

> *No man ever steps in the same river twice,*
> *for it's not the same river and he's not the*
> *same man.*
>
> *- Heraclitus*

Only the flexible survive!

When it comes to dealing with the rapid change of a crisis – a pandemic, a war, a global disaster – it's not always the strong that survive. Flexibility and adaptability become even more critical factors. The most powerful muscles in our body are not just strong, they are flexible and resist becoming tied up in a knot from stress.

Experts agree that our ability to stay present enhances our chances of navigating a crisis successfully. Disaster expert Anie Kalayjian says, *"Being in the moment does not mean being unaware of the consequences of any actions you take; it means you do not have a prejudgment about those consequences. As a result,"* she says, *"it keeps us from panicking over what could possibly happen and allows us to stay focused on what is happening."*

In the same light, Dr. Al Siebert, author of **The Resiliency Advantage** , says *"the best survivors are the ones who are able to "read" the new reality rapidly, focus on problem solving, and take practical action – all within the moment. There's a fair amount of flexibility needed – the personality who can adapt quickly to changes and feel certain about their ability to do so is usually the type that handles a crisis well."*

Resilience is defined as the ability to flexibly adapt to challenging, adverse, or traumatic life events. Resilience is not a trait that you either have or do not have; rather, it is a set of strategies that can be learned and practiced.

- Arielle Schwartz@ProjectHappines_org

It is the same with our emotional and mental toughness. Whether working with seasoned executives or young athletes, we have experienced firsthand the importance of emotional and mental toughness and resilience in achieving success. High-performing individuals and teams work to strengthen their bodies and their minds in preparation for weathering seasons of adversity. This kind of toughness is deeply rooted in their personal values and team culture and they understand the benefit of using the wind to power their efforts instead of resisting what they cannot control.

The Oak Tree and the Palm Tree

If asked, *"Which would you rather be, an Oak Tree or a Palm Tree?"* many of us would choose the Oak. Oak trees are known for being strong and sturdy, with deep roots and a commanding presence. Palm trees, on the other hand, are slender, tall, and beautiful, but appear to sway in even the slightest breeze. What most people don't realize about Palm trees is that their roots also run deep.

When faced with adversity, many people would want to have the strength and sturdiness of the Oak tree. However, let's think about what happens in a storm. Due to their solid, unmovable nature, Oak trees are often uprooted or broken by high winds and heavy rain. The Palm tree, however, leans and sways in the direction of the wind – knowing that it's better to go with the force of a great storm than against it. Without the pressure of resisting the wind, the heavy rain nourishes and deepens the roots of the Palm, preparing it to weather the next storm. Although the palm tree might be stripped of its fronds for a few months after a storm, the tree survives and the fronds re-grow, as beautiful as ever!

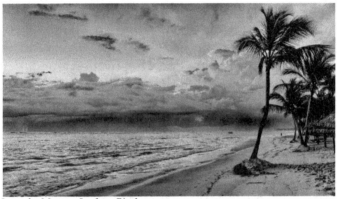

Image by MustangJoe from Pixabay

Re-prioritize what matters most

If anything, COVID-19 has forced us to look at our priorities and what matters most to us. The mandated changes to our everyday life have forced us to find ways to cope and keep moving forward. More people are tele-commuting and working from home. Kids are learning remotely. Delivery has become the new "night out". We are re-discovering our favorite books, movies, and board games, not to mention our loved ones.

Although there are serious implications to so many industries, especially with the closure of non-essential businesses, entrepreneurs everywhere are overcoming their initial shock and finding ways to serve. Restaurants are now only open for delivery and pick up. Businesses are using virtual workplaces for their teams to collaborate. Schools are delivering lessons through e-learning. The Internet has become once again a place that connects us. Social media is being used to stay connected with loved ones and support each other, rather than a way to compare and contrast views and lifestyles.

It's easy to panic and empty the shelves at the store, desperately trying to hoard toilet paper and hand sanitizer. But once we get over the initial fears and look around, we realize what's important to us. When we accept that this is not going to be over in a few days or a week, that this temporary inconvenience may be something more permanent, we can adjust our thinking to a "new normal."

Nothing more permanent than the temporary.

- Greek Proverb

University of Adversity

We all must deal with troubles at one time or another. None of us will pass through this mortal existence unscathed. Part of the human experience is to face challenges and trials. If they are faced with courage and faith, they can help us to grow in ways that nothing else can.

A smooth sea never made a skillful mariner.

- Unknown

Most of us don't see adversity as a blessing. We fight it, we hate it, we worry about it, and we stress over it. However, adversity makes us stronger and more compassionate towards others experiencing trials; it makes us wiser and helps us appreciate life more. There is opposition in all aspects of this life. But that opposition can also help us to recognize our blessings. Without sadness, we wouldn't recognize joy. Without pain, we wouldn't understand pleasure. After illness, we appreciate much more our good health. Nobody escapes this life with only "smooth sailing." And it's important to recognize the times when we are experiencing "smooth sailing" to appreciate them.

Can we be happy while we're suffering? The truth is, yes, we can. If we waited for the perfect day when every conflict was resolved, every debt was repaid, and every problem was eliminated, then we would have put off happiness indefinitely. There is a point to the adversity in our lives, because what "doesn't kill us" truly does make us stronger. If we choose to grow from our setbacks, we will be prepared to meet other disappointments with greater peace and optimism. We will be blessed with greater compassion, and those insights that will allow us to help others facing similar situations. If we use the adversity in our lives to our advantage, it absolutely can be a positive thing.

If we can recognize the positive events going on in our lives while we're in the middle of a challenge, we will overcome the experience feeling peace, rather than worry or stress.

Adversity and pain have a way of crystalizing our thoughts and helping us zoom in to what's really important to us. They help us peel away the layers of wants to get to the true needs. From there we can seek new and meaningful life-choices as we go beyond just surviving.

Improvise, adapt, and overcome!

Points to Ponder:

Adversity can help us grow stronger, to deepen our roots.

- Strength is important, but flexibility is essential as life is unpredictable.

- Keep an open mind and cultivate the ability to adapt in any situation.

Questions to Consider:

- Can you identify what triggers you to be in a particular mode? Complete the following sentences:

    a. I tend to feel like a Victim when…

    b. I tend to feel like a Critic when…

    c. I tend to feel like a Bystander when…

    d. I tend to feel like a Navigator when…

- What will help you move to a more (emotionally) productive place? (Hint: It might be addressing your triggers for unproductive behaviors)

- What have you always wanted to do but felt you never had the time? Use the answer to this question and start working on your dream.

Take Action:

- List all the areas that you are holding on too tight and refusing to change.

- Which ones do you need to show flexibility in?

- How will you use your flexibility to form a solution?

Key #4: Preparation

Part of the problem we face in trying to handle stress, is that most of us are constantly operating in crisis-management mode rather than taking a proactive approach to our lives. We feel like we are continually putting out fires, going from one thing to the next. Can you visualize yourself going through life carrying a fire extinguisher all the time? Putting out fires to the left, to the right, above and below you? That's no way to live! Living in a reactive mode will never bring peace of mind or happiness.

> *Maintaining order rather than correcting disorder is the ultimate principle of wisdom. To cure disease after it has appeared is like digging a well when one feels thirsty, or forging weapons after the war has already begun.*
>
> *Nei Jing, 2nd century BC*

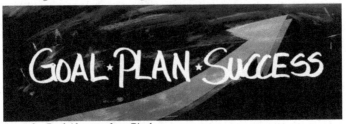

Image by Gerd Altmann from Pixabay

Operate in Prevention Mode.

Crisis *prevention* is the key because it's less expensive financially, physically, emotionally and mentally than crisis *management*. This is true regarding every aspect of our lives. Wouldn't it be better for us to change some habits now, like eating healthier and exercising, rather than waiting for a crisis, such as a heart attack, to hit and force us to make those changes? What about learning to live within our means with an actual budget, rather than accumulating debt, which could lead us to bankruptcy.

Consider all the unnecessary emotional and mental stress we're putting ourselves through by not acting on our issues before they get out of control. Most things in life can be prevented if we take the time to address them. We're all familiar with POST Traumatic Stress Disorder or PTSD. We'd like to introduce the concept of **PRE-Traumatic Stress (Pre-TS):** the tension, anxiety, and stress we experience when we anticipate a traumatic event, when we are bracing for the impact it will have on us and our lives. Anyone that has been in a car accident, can certainly relate to the feeling of bracing before impact. This can be so powerful for many of us that it can paralyze us, confuse our thinking, and fill us with despair before anything has even happened. It can move us to an unproductive place and not allow us to act in a way that will prepare us for what we must do next.

Emotional Preparedness

Taking care of our emotional health may be the single most important factor to how well we weather any crisis that we may face. It is natural to feel stress, anxiety, grief, and worry before, during, and after a disaster. Everyone reacts differently, and our feelings will most likely change over time. Consciously becoming aware of our feelings and accepting them for what they are will go a long way to overcoming our fears. Taking care of our emotional health before, as well as during, an emergency will help us think clearly and react to the urgent needs to protect ourselves, our loved ones and those less fortunate than us. Self-care during an unforeseen crisis will also contribute to our long-term healing.

There are several ways we can cope better as events beyond our control, at times frightening and unexpected, unfold before us.

We can plan to:

- **Connect with others** – At a time of crisis it becomes imperative to access our support system. Especially if sheltering in place, being quarantined, following social distancing is required, we still need to connect with others. If we're not physically able to connect with our support system, we can always reach out via a phone call, text, or social media. Now more than ever, it's time to be real, to allow ourselves to be vulnerable and honest. Sharing our concerns and how we're feeling with a friend, family member, or a trusted advisor can make all the difference during a crisis.

- **Take breaks** – During the COVID-19 pandemic most of us found ourselves with plenty of time on our hands. This may be a unique characteristic of this crisis, as in

- other situations we might be running for our lives (literally!). For many this was a time of great distress but also an opportunity to alter our "rat-race" mentality. To switch from living as human-doings and becoming human beings! Think about that for a minute. Which would you rather be? We realize a lot of people's self-worth comes from the human-doing side but also most of the stress and anxiety comes from it as well. Living more frequently as a human being has brought more peace and greater happiness. It has felt good to eat together, play together, and work together side by side as families and loved ones. So be mindful of your energy levels, and plan for physical and mental breaks in your day.

- **Stay informed** – It is not unusual to feel that we are missing information or not getting the whole truth from official sources, government entities at the local, state, or even national level. This may create additional stress and feelings of impending doom. We fear the unknown and too often create scenarios in our minds which end up being far worse than the reality on the ground. In the age of "fake" news, conspiracy theories, and fearmongering, it is important to check our sources. Be aware that there may be rumors during a crisis, especially on social media. Watch, listen to, or read the news for updates from officials. Always check our inflow of communication and turn to reliable sources of information. If they have been trustworthy in the past the likelihood is that they will tell you the truth now. It's also important to check our sources before passing on the information to others. The last things we want to do is spread false rumors!

- **Avoid too much exposure to news** – It may seem entirely contradictory from staying informed as stated above, but we also need to take breaks from watching, reading, or listening to news stories. There is a balancing act that we must achieve because it can be upsetting to hear about the crisis, the loss of lives, and see images of destruction repeatedly. The number of deaths and destruction can be staggering, especially if the crisis is ongoing like the pandemic. The grim news every hour of every single day can numb the senses and overwhelm even the most positive person among us. It's good to stay informed but it's unhealthy to keep getting hourly notifications or "breaking news" which are merely repetitions of what we already know.

- **Have enjoyable moments** – It's important to fill our time, even under quarantine and "sheltering in place" with activities we enjoy. Reading a good book, binge-watching a favorite series, or just exercising our body and mind at home can help significantly. Interestingly, many parents are reporting the joy of rediscovering playing with their children, using chalk to draw positive images and messages with them on sidewalks, or just reconnecting through fun activities. Adults playing cards and board games and socializing with each other. Communications in the form of in-depth discussions about the meaning of life or the way we wish to live in the future seem to dominate many households. These are some of the blessings in disguise that have arisen as we all have been forced to hunker down together. Wherever possible, going out for walks in nature or around our neighborhoods have also increased. Of course, we still need to abide by the social distancing parameters that are set in order to keep us all safe.

- **Seek help when needed** – When crises or unforeseen events last from a few days to weeks or months at a time then distress, depression or worse can set in. It's quite normal to desire to have our lives return to what we had before. However, the "new normal" may end up becoming the new normal so there's a need for us to adjust. If we for whatever reason begin to have of daily life or activities be negatively impacted by the seemingly never-ending stress, then it's ok to seek professional assistance. Whether it's talking to our doctor, counselor, or member of the clergy, know that such reaching out is healthy and a big part of staying emotionally on top of things.

These planning ideas have shown to be invaluable for reducing the personal stress or even trauma people have experienced when the emergency period is prolonged. It's not uncommon following a crisis for the recovery period to take weeks or months before things return to "normal". However, in the case of the COVID-19 Pandemic, the duration of the crisis alone that cost so many lives, closed so many businesses, and forced many emergency measures, has been significant! It can feel at times like a prolonged "battle" or "war zone", and perhaps explains why some even characterize this crisis as "humanity's war against a silent but deadly enemy".

Assess the (potential) impact of the crisis

Beyond the emotional preparedness, there are probably some very practical considerations we will need to address. If we take the time to look at how the crisis may – potentially but realistically – impact us, we will be in a better position to see likely problem areas and take appropriate steps to prepare. This honest look can also help us make the most of our ability to adapt successfully to necessary changes, while reducing the emotional distress and discomfort that crises bring.

To accomplish this, we first need good information – perhaps from multiple sources or perspectives – so we can best determine how the crisis will affect (or is affecting) us and others. We can then pull together the information in a way that will help us understand and act on it. Depending on our preferences, we may want to create a simple list, outline, or even a drawing that shows how we are being or will be affected. Especially when working on a plan with others (i.e. family members, partners, dependents, etc.), summarizing the information we've gathered will help us evaluate things, identify ways to overcome problems, and make appropriate choices about how to move forward. We cannot rely simply on "luck", and "hope" is not really an effective strategy. Successfully navigating a crisis requires planning and preparation to minimize missteps and overcome the problems that will inevitably arise.

Luck is what happens when preparation meets opportunity.

- Seneca

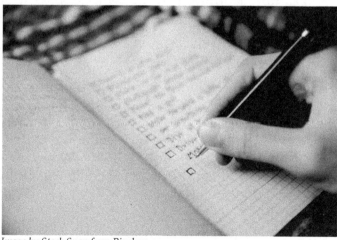

Image by Stock Snap from Pixabay

How ready are you for an emergency?

Preparation is a key to success regardless of the type of challenges we're facing. In sports, the championship teams of lore, or the elite athletes that dominate their respective sport, always out-prepare their opponents. The same holds true for the game called life! And preparation becomes even more of a necessity when we are dealing with crises like natural disasters or pandemics. Preparedness could literally save our life and the lives of our loved ones.

A great resource for preparedness planning is **Ready.gov**, an official website of the Department of Homeland Security that outlines emergency preparedness information during a variety of crises. The site also has links to the **Federal Emergency Management Agency (FEMA)** and the **Centers for Disease Control and Prevention (CDC)** websites with relevant information*.

> *****Note:** For those readers outside the U.S.A., please refer to your country's official agencies.

Here is an **example from the website** with helpful information and considerations about what to do <u>before</u> a Pandemic:

- Store additional supplies of food and water.

- Periodically check your regular prescription drugs to ensure a continuous supply in your home.

- Have any nonprescription drugs and other health supplies on hand, including pain relievers, stomach remedies, cough and cold medicines, fluids with electrolytes, and vitamins.

- Get copies and maintain electronic versions of health records from doctors, hospitals, pharmacies and other sources and store them, for personal reference. Get help accessing **electronic health records.**

- Talk with family members and loved ones about how they would be cared for if they got sick, or what will be needed to care for them in your home. Depending on the type of emergency or crisis, it is important to note the two prevailing strategies: Shelter in Place, as we are facing during this pandemic, and Getting Mobile.

Shelter in Place

Recent guidance is clear about the need for people to **shelter in place**. For those feeling anxious it might help to think about potential challenges and make a plan for them. Here are some practical considerations:

- **Supplies:** Think about how you could get any supplies you need – either from a delivery service, a neighbor, family, or friends so you don't have to worry about running out. Try to pick healthy food, especially as you might not get as much exercise as normal.

- **Cash:** If possible, it's a good idea to have at least the equivalent of one or two paychecks in cash stored at home for any emergency conditions, or if access to your bank or an ATM is restricted.

- **Financial concerns:** You may be worried about work and money if you have to stay home – these issues can have a big impact on your mental health. For guidance on what your rights are at work, what benefits you are entitled, and what further support is available, contact your organization's Human Resources department. If you are self-employed, check reputable sources such as

- your industry's association, your Chamber of Commerce, or other government agencies for the latest details.

- **If you are being treated for existing conditions:** Continue accessing treatment and support where possible. Let relevant services know that you are staying at home and work out how to continue receiving support during this time. Consider having appointments with your doctor, nurse, counselor, or other caretaker by phone, text, or online. If any of your needed health care services will be affected by staying at home, let your providers know so alternative arrangements can be put in place.

- **If you are taking medication(s) for existing conditions:** Most pharmacies now offer auto-refill prescriptions by phone, or online. A good idea might be to ask your pharmacy about getting your medication delivered or think about who you could ask to collect it for you.

- **If you care for other people:** You may be worried about how to ensure care for those who rely on you – either your dependents at home or others that you regularly visit. Special accommodations are being put in place by companies, as well as state governments to help caretakers under these extreme and prolonged conditions. Extra planning may be required for those providing care or supporting someone they don't live with.

Getting Mobile

If we need to get mobile because of hurricanes, earthquakes, floods, fires, or other natural disasters, then it would be a good idea to have a **72-hour Emergency Kit**. For a good example, access Ready.gov, for details and guidelines.

The website provides practical advice on preparing, storing, and maintaining your **72-hour Emergency Kit**. The page includes important information on the things needed in an emergency, such as water, food, first-aid, cash, and simple items to help create a basic shelter. It also includes items that might be less obvious, like a radio, a flashlight, extra batteries, a can opener, and local maps. We've become accustomed to using our cell phones for everything, but what if we can't charge our phones or access a functioning network in a disaster? Depending on your unique needs and your surrounding environment, it will make sense to download **the detailed list** from the website and personalize your preparation to fit your particular situation.

Points to Ponder:

- Manage your Pre-TS emotions to free your thinking and actions.

- Choose prevention over crisis management.

- Preparedness is key to successfully navigating any crisis.

Questions to Consider:

What do <u>you</u> need to do to prepare for an emergency?

- If you are asked to Shelter in Place, do you have enough food, supplies, and cash to survive as a family, or at least access to those essentials?

- If you need to Get Mobile, do you have a 72-Hour Emergency Kit for yourself and each member of your family?

Take Action:

- Create a list of potential needs you (and your family) will have in an emergency or crisis.

- Identify any problem areas you will need to address or questions you still need to answer.

- Create your plan to address those outstanding items.

Key #5: Initiative

The difference between who you are and who you want to be is what you do.

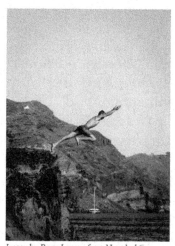
Image by Roan Lavery from Unsplash

In the previous chapter we discussed different way to prepare ourselves and others for life-changing events. We may not always have advanced notice before a specific event, but our preparation can serve us well, nonetheless. In this chapter, we will look at ways to put our plan into action and reclaim some control where we can.

The ability to take action is a very empowering feeling. When we feel we can act on a problem to solve it, or simply improve a situation, we feel better about ourselves and more confident about our ability to overcome our challenges. That in turn has a positive impact on our attitude and allows us to feel better about taking the next step, and then the next step. And with each step, we gain valuable momentum that can help us overcome adversity. The key is our willingness and ability to take the initiative and to move forward.

> *Even if you're on the right track, you'll get run over if you just sit there.*
>
> *- Will Rogers*

Fear is a natural emotional response to a crisis. Fear can mobilize us to act: to fight or run ... but too much fear can actually paralyze us. Some will begin this movement sooner than others; they will find the strength and desire to act and do what must be done. Others need more time, more encouragement, and more support to take action. That's OK! We can help each other overcome the hesitation and inertia caused by fear.

Our actions can also inspire others to act. When the NBA made the difficult decision to suspend the season, a number of the league's star players such as Kevin Love and Giannis Antetokounmpo donated money to pay for the salaries of hourly arena workers that would be directly impacted by the closures. Shortly after that, team owners like Arthur Blank stepped up and committed to covering those lost hourly wages for employees. Following their example, many other professional players and owners of teams have committed to contribute financially and provide compassionate support to the many anonymous and vulnerable workers (and their families) that are impacted by the pandemic and are in jeopardy of losing their health and their livelihood.

Start simple

When we're dealing with a crisis or major event, it's normal to feel a loss of control. We shouldn't expect to be able to take on everything at once. Instead, we can take charge of what we <u>can</u> do and encourage others to do the same. Consider the following ideas as a starting point:

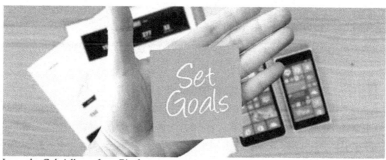

Image by Gabrielle_cc from Pixabay

- **Set goals:** Setting goals and achieving them gives a sense of control and purpose – think about things you want or need to do that you can still do at home. It could be finishing a project, watching a film, reading a book, or learning something online.

- **Keep your mind active:** Read, write, play games, do crossword puzzles, sudokus, jigsaws or drawing and painting. Find something that works for you.

- **Take time to relax and focus on the present:** This can help with difficult emotions, worries about the future, and can improve wellbeing. Relaxation techniques can also help some people to deal with feelings of anxiety. Here's a **simple idea from the Mayo Clinic Health System staff.**

  Sit quietly. Look around you and notice:
  - 5 things you can see: Your hands, the sky, a plant on a nearby table.

- 4 things you can physically feel: Your feet on the ground, a ball, your friend's hand.

- 3 things you can hear: The wind blowing, children's laughter, your breath.

- 2 things you can smell: Fresh-cut grass, coffee, soap.

- 1 thing you can taste: A mint, gum, the fresh air.

This exercise helps you shift your focus to your surroundings in the present moment and away from what is causing you to feel anxious. It can help interrupt unhealthy thought patterns.

- **If you can, once a day get outside, or bring nature in:** Spending time in green spaces can benefit both our mental and physical wellbeing. If we can't get outside much we can try to still get these positive effects by spending time with the windows open to let in fresh air, arranging space to sit and see a nice view (if possible) and get some natural sunlight, or get out into the garden if we can.

We should remember that social distancing guidelines enable us to go outside, as long as we are careful and keep 6 feet apart from others who are not members of our household.

What can help our mental health and wellbeing?

If we can't do the things we normally enjoy because we're staying home, we can still try to think about how we could adapt them or try something new. There are lots of free tutorials and courses online and people are coming up with innovative online solutions like online coffee chats and streamed live music concerts. People are gathering virtually in small and large groups to connect and share experiences in very unique and innovative ways.

- **Reach out to our loved ones:** Maintaining our connection with the important people in our life is important for our mental health and wellbeing. We can seek ways to stay in touch with friends and family via telephone, video calls, texting, or social media, whether it's people we see regularly or (re)connecting with old friends.

- **Talk about our concerns:** It's quite common to feel worried, scared or helpless about our current situation. Keep in mind that this is a difficult time for everyone and sharing how we are feeling and the things we are doing to cope with family and friends can help them too. We can also consider talking to a mental health professional, or we could find support groups online to join.

- **Help and support others:** We can think about how we could help those around us – it will make a big difference to them and can make us feel better too. Perhaps we could message a friend or family member just to check in with them, join a community group to (safely) support others locally, offer to help our older friends and neighbors with their grocery shopping, or thank one of the many doctors, nurses, delivery people, policemen/women, and others who are working so tirelessly to support and safeguard us during this time.

- **Look after our physical wellbeing:** Our physical health has a big impact on how we feel emotionally and mentally. At times of crisis, it can be easy to fall into unhealthy patterns of behavior, which in turn can make us feel worse. Instead we can make an extra effort to eat healthy, well-balanced meals, drink plenty of water, exercise inside where possible, get outside once a day, and try to avoid smoking, alcohol, and drugs.

(Coach Kon) My daughter spends large parts of her day in front of a computer, completing her school assignments like so many other students. She uses her wearable health tracker to remind her to move. I watch her at least once an hour get up and say, "It's Walk O'clock dad!" and walk around the house to get her target steps in. She is an inspiration to me to stay active.

If we can go outside, we can walk, run, hike, or garden (always following the recommended social distancing guidelines). If that's not an option and we are forced to stay inside, there are plenty of exercise videos and challenges online to try at home, or we can get creative and play ping-pong on our dining room table, set up a "home Olympics course", or make up our own fun ideas to stay active.

- **Look after our sleep:** Good-quality sleep makes a big difference to how we feel mentally and physically, so it's important to get enough. However, feeling anxious or worried can make it harder to get a good night's sleep. To make it easier, to maintain regular sleeping patterns, while at the same time avoiding (electronic) screens before bed, cutting back on caffeine, and creating a restful environment.

- **Try to manage difficult feelings:** Many people find the news about coronavirus (COVID-19) concerning. However, some people may experience such intense anxiety that it becomes a problem. It's okay to acknowledge that some things are outside our control right now, but constant repetitive thoughts about the situation, which can lead some to feel anxious, overwhelmed, or even helpless, are not healthy. Instead, we can try to focus on the things we can control. If the difficult feelings continue, we should consider getting more information on how to manage anxiety, or even consult a health professional.

- **Manage our media and information intake:** Round the clock news and constant social media updates can make us more worried. If we feel negatively affected, we can try to limit the time we spend watching, reading, or listening to media coverage of the crisis. It may help to only check the news at set times or limiting to a couple of checks a day.

- **Get the facts:** Gather factual information that will help accurately determine our own or other people's risk of contracting coronavirus (COVID-19) so that we can take reasonable precautions. Find a credible source we can trust, such as the **Centers for Disease Control and Prevention website**, and fact check information that we get from newsfeeds, social media, or from other people. We should also avoid sharing information without fact-checking it against credible sources. Passing on inaccurate information during fearful times can be especially harmful.

- **Think about our new daily routine:** Life is changing for us all for a while. Whether we are staying at home or social distancing, we are likely to see some disruption to our normal routine. This is an opportunity for us to think about how we can adapt and create positive new routines – try to engage in useful activities (such as cleaning, cooking or exercise) or meaningful activities (such as reading or calling a friend). We might find it helpful to write a plan for your day or your week.

- **Do things we enjoy:** To counteract our feelings of anxiety, loneliness, or sadness we can try things that lift our spirits. Focusing on our favorite hobby, learning something new, or simply taking time to relax indoors should give us some relief from anxious thoughts and feelings, and can boost our mood. A simple afternoon nap can help us feel refreshed and rejuvenated.

I am not what has happened to me. I am
what I choose to become.

- Carl Jung

Bringing our work(place) home

Working from home may not be a new experience for many of us. Before the spread of the coronavirus, roughly half of American workers were doing at least some telework. For many of us that can still perform our job remotely, the transition may seem simple, but it's not easy! Working remotely full-time forces us to look at our work and productivity very differently. We quickly discover that things we took for granted previously in the office, such as easy access to equipment, resources, and people, may require us to get creative, think differently, and be more flexible and patient with ourselves and others.

So, how can we continue to be productive during this time with so many things competing for our attention? How can we find the right balance between life and work and fit it all in a single space?

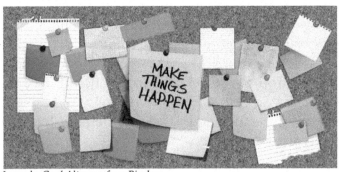

Image by Gerd Altmann from Pixabay

Some of the requirements of a home office are obvious. For example, a computer with access to the right technology can minimize the distance between us and our regular office and team as we work virtually. With high speed access to the internet, we can participate in all the video conferencing, number crunching, and file sharing we need to get the job done.

If more than one person is working (or learning) from home, however, it's critical to set up a plan to accommodate everyone's needs. With multiple working adults, each will need to find an appropriate space to do his or her work. If there are children in the house, will they need to do schoolwork, to be supervised, entertained, or otherwise engaged? Who will be responsible? Can we find the time and space to handle work responsibilities, while also accommodating and supporting the needs of others? We may need to compromise and take turns, share a table or work area, and be even more flexible with our schedule. We also need to be patient with ourselves and our family members when those things we had planned to accomplish, didn't quite get done.

Separating work time and personal time is much harder when working from home. Getting dressed in the morning as if going into the office, can trigger a more professional behavior and mindset. It's also important to set time boundaries for lunch, breaks, and the end of the "work" day. Getting up and walking around at least once an hour and tackling work in blocks or chunks of similar activities, are simple things we can do to help us stay productive. Over time, the lines between our personal and work time can get very blurry, making it harder to focus on each and still be effective in the same space.

The best thing we can do for our mental health and wellbeing is to be kind to ourselves and others, remembering that during difficult times, it's normal if we're not accomplishing what we normally might be able to … stress takes a huge mental and emotional toll.

Take Action Individually and with Others

For all these changes and adjustments to be successful, the people involved need to take responsibility for their success.
We can take stock of what needs to get done during this time and agree on the best order to do things. Developing a shared plan and goals enables everyone to work together to make the most of the situation. This can involve family, partners, coworkers, clients, etc. working together to agree on what can and cannot be done during this time. We may all believe things will return to "normal" soon, but in the meantime clear expectations and communication will help prevent problems.

Being a navigator during a crisis does not always mean looking at the positive side. We also need to be aware of where the plan may not be working. We must remain alert to changes that need to be made and to ways that may no longer be effective because of the new conditions and limitations. For example, if we can't get to the store, can we order products to be delivered? If we can't meet in person, can we find a collaborative platform online to work together? As consultants, we have been working and teaching remotely with our clients and partners – and it's getting easier the more we use the available tools.

> *When we focus on ourselves, our world contracts as our problems loom large. But when we focus on others, our world expands.*
>
> *Daniel Goleman*

Frustration with the necessary changes during a crisis often comes from not looking past the obstacles they present. Instead of getting mired in the negatives, we can try to stay focused on the broader, societal need or greater good that's driving and necessitating the changes. We can encourage others to do the same. This will help us not only remain objective about the situation, but also maintain positive relationships. It is not unreasonable to feel the personal discomfort of the changes and initially resist. But it's important to keep our "eye on the prize". The inconvenience is temporary while the gains will be lasting.

If following safety guidelines will keep us and our loved ones safe, then it's a small price to pay. We may be required to keep a safe "social distance" from each other, but we can still have honest conversations. We may not see each other every day in person, but we can talk over the phone or video chat. Restaurants may not be able to serve patrons in their store, but they are able to keep their doors open for delivery and pickup. The pain we feel now is temporary, and things <u>will</u> get better!

During the upheaval of a crisis, everybody makes mistakes. That's one thing we can count on. However, we can set an example for others by taking our own mistakes in stride. It is only by making mistakes that we – and others – will find a way to get through the difficult times successfully, as long as we learn from them. It's important to remember that successful people make as many mistakes as everyone else. What differentiates them are the following 3 characteristics:

1. They own their mistakes by taking personal responsibility. Successful people are not victims of their choices nor do they blame others or circumstances for their failures. They stand up, look in the mirror and say "Yep, that's on me. Nobody forced me to make that decision. I own it!"

2. They learn their lessons and don't continue to repeat their mistakes. It has been said that there are no true failures in life: people either win, or they learn. As long as they continue to learn from their choices and their consequences, they are moving forward.

3. They let them go and move on! By forgiving themselves quickly and often they move on in life to bigger and better things! They don't carry with them the "dead weight" of disappointment, discouragement and resentment. In essence, they are free, unencumbered by past choices and actually emboldened to do better based on the lessons learned.

Working in the Danger Zone

But what about the remaining third of American workers that cannot work remotely — food service, construction, and factory workers, people who are stocking the shelves in grocery stores and warehouses, police officers and fire fighters, nurses and doctors on the front lines of health care? They can't work from home.

Despite the advances of technology, some jobs require workers to be physically present. If we really can't work remotely, we can ask our employer what we can do to make sure we are safe, while preserving our income. It's not clear that hourly workers or workers who can't do remote work will be paid if they can't work. Recently, governments across the globe have begun compensating workers that are forced to stay home due to the circumstances and the direct impact of the pandemic on their jobs and industry. The number of people that have been laid off due to the forced closure of businesses are in the millions, and they are being supported in the short-term through enhanced unemployment benefits.

As we lose ourselves in the service of others, we discover our own lives and our own happiness.

Dieter f. Uchtdorf

In some cases, the entrepreneurial spirit is making progress and overcoming adversity through innovation and creativity. Businesses are finding new ways to deliver their services and products. New industries are flourishing as other, more traditional ones are being forced dormant. This upheaval has opened up new frontiers, and the thought that we will ever go back to "business as usual" may be a pipedream for many. The possibility of a global pandemic and its impact is no longer a hypothetical; it is already here!

Points to Ponder:

The difference between who you are and who you want to be is what you do.

- Take positive action individually and with others to make things better.

- When making a mistake remember the 3 steps for success: Own it, learn from it, and let it go!

Questions to Consider:

What's your plan of action during this time?

- What specific actions can you take individually? When?

- What specific actions can you take with others? When?

Take Action:

- Enter the answers from the above Questions to Consider in the space provided below.

- Write a date next to each action to indicate when you plan to do it. (This will add a sense of urgency and focus to help you complete the tasks)

Individual Actions   Date

_____

_____

_____

_____

Actions with Others   Date

_____

_____

_____

_____

Key #6: Positive Attitude

Dr. Viktor Frankl, the bestselling author of "Man's Search for Meaning" and a renowned Austrian psychiatrist, survived the Holocaust in Germany. While watching his fellow inmates in a Nazi concentration camp, he observed that "all things could be taken from a man except the final freedom: the ability to choose how he will respond to any situation." When visiting the Auschwitz concentration camp where Dr. Frankl was an inmate, the strength of the human spirit and the profound truth of his observations strike with a stunning force.

Are You an Optimist or a Pessimist?

As we grow up and learn from those around us, and as we experience the events that occur in our lives, we may allow the lens through which we view the world to become warped - too focused on the negative. Do you see the glass half full, or half empty? What is the real difference between being an optimist vs. being a pessimist?

*A pessimist sees the difficulty in every
opportunity; an optimist sees the
opportunity in every difficulty.*

— Sir Winston Churchill

There's an anecdote that illustrates the point well: the optimist wakes up every morning, looks out the window and says, "Good morning, Lord!" Before anything else takes place, there's an acknowledgement and expression of gratitude to start off the day. The pessimist wakes up the same morning, looks out the same window and declares, "Good Lord, it's morning!" Clearly, nothing bad has transpired yet, but there's already lament for the new day ahead. So, the day begins and they're both wearing their expectations on their sleeves.
Everything that will take place during the day will be viewed through their unique lens.

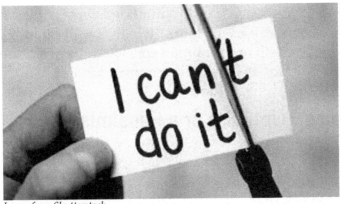
Image from Shutterstock

Imagine the following example: both the optimist and the pessimist get a flat tire on the way to work as they're exiting the freeway, but they have different reactions. The optimist counts his blessings because the flat happened as the car was slowing down on the exit ramp, and not while it was traveling on the freeway at 70 miles per hour. Gratitude fills his heart for being so fortunate! The pessimist pulls over, inspects the flat tire and thinks to himself, "Why do these things always happen to me? Now I'll be late for work and my boss will probably fire me!"

In my experience, it is also impossible to feel depressed or upset when we are focusing on those blessings we are grateful for. Try it! Next time you are feeling anxious or down, take ten minutes and begin listing everything you can think of, for which you are grateful (name individual friends and family members, your five senses, your home, the freedom you enjoy, health, nature, love, work, etc., and let that gratitude sink deep down into your soul as you picture and think of each item. After ten minutes, your mindset should be in a much better place!

People who are pessimists ask questions like, "What's wrong with my life . . . my parents . . . my kids . . . my spouse?" Anybody who actually asks those questions out loud will get very long responses, especially to that last one! When negative questions are asked, negativity rules! But if we ask positive questions instead, such as:

- What am I grateful for?

- Who loves me?

- What's great about my family?

- What can I do today to make someone happy?

- What do I admire about my husband / wife?

Then the focus of the lens through which we view life will change, and we can become an optimist.

What if...?

In a time of crisis, it's more than likely we can find many negative examples simply due to the nature of the situation. Finding positives however is much harder, but it's important nonetheless to attempt. What if we changed the way we asked the questions? What if we looked for the light in the darkness, the silver lining? During the Coronavirus Pandemic, we received the following poetic message from a loved one:

> *There is so much fear, and perhaps rightfully so,*
> *about COVID-19.*
>
> *And, what if...*
>
> *If we subscribe to the philosophy that life is always*
> *working out for us, that there is an intelligence far*
> *greater than humans at work...*
>
> *That all is interconnected.*
>
> *What if...*
>
> *the virus is here to help us?*
>
> *To reset.*
>
> *To remember.*
>
> *What is truly important.*
>
> *Reconnecting with family and community.*
>
> *Reducing travel so that the environment, the skies,*
> *the air, our lungs all get a break.*

Parts of China are seeing blue sky and clouds for the first time in forever with the factories being shut down.

Working from home rather than commuting to work (less pollution, more personal time).

Reconnecting with family as there is more time at home.

An invitation to turn inwards — a deep meditation — rather than the usual extroverted going out to self-soothe.

To reconnect with self — what is really important to me?

A reset economically.

The working poor. The lack of healthcare access for over 30 million in the US. The need for paid sick leave.

How hard does one need to work to be able to live, to have a life outside of work?

To face our mortality — check back into "living" life rather than simply working, working, working.

To reconnect with our elders, who are so susceptible to this virus.

And, washing our hands — how did that become a "new" thing that we needed to remember. But, yes, we did.

The presence of Grace for all.

There is a shift underway in our society — what if it is one that is favorable for us?

What if this virus is an ally in our evolution?

In our remembrance of what it means to be connected, humane, living a simpler life, to be less impactful/ more kind to our environment.

An offering from my heart this morning. Offered as another perspective. Another way of relating to this virus, this unfolding, this evolution.

It was time for a change, we all knew that.

And, change has arrived.

What if...

(Attributed to Gutpreet K. Gill)

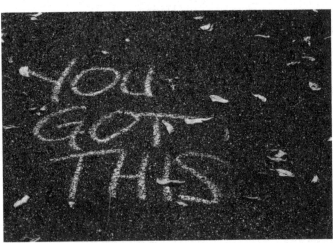

Image by Sydney Rae from Unsplash

Avoid comparisons

Another attribute that commonly appears during a crisis, making comparisons. Any limitations and restrictions that are put in place can create a "scarcity mindset" for many, and trigger an almost primal sense of competition and a survival instinct that makes us feel like "there is not enough to go around." We tell ourselves, "I have to secure enough for myself and my family." "What if (whatever resource we value) runs out?" And then we are panic-buying toilet paper, hand sanitizer, and frozen pizza!

We look at other peoples' shopping carts and feel we don't have enough. We talk to friends and neighbors and evaluate how well we've prepared for the crisis. "Has John got more supplies in his garage than me?" "How come Suzy's kids are so well prepared to study at home?" "Why didn't I think of stocking up on popcorn and ice cream?" Every time we compare ourselves to another person, there are only two possible outcomes:

1. Either we'll decide "I'm better than you are," and then we're guilty of being arrogant and prideful, or

2. We'll conclude, "You're better than I am," which makes us feel bad about ourselves – like we're not good enough.

Most people engage in such comparisons, and frequently with unpleasant results. Who doesn't know an arrogant person who thinks he's better than everybody else? Ironically, this kind of behavior stems from insecurity. A person who brags has a little voice inside himself or herself saying, "I'm not good enough – I have to prove myself."

It really doesn't make any sense for us to compare ourselves to other people. Whether it's financially, spiritually, emotionally, physically, or something else – we will never be on exactly the same level as anybody else. There will always be somebody thinner, richer, more prepared or smarter than we are, and likewise, there will always be somebody who's less attractive, less financially successful, less prepared or less educated. If we spend our time "tooting our own horn" to let others know how great we are, we're not impressing anyone – we're really quite annoying! And every time we compare ourselves to others and fall short, we're making a withdrawal from our "self-worth account." Sometimes a lack of self-worth can lead to indulgence in destructive habits as we try to find comfort, such as excessive eating or shopping, or even the abuse of drugs or alcohol. Ironically, the things we turn to for comfort actually damage us even more, especially if we develop an addiction. So, how do we stop ourselves from engaging in this unpleasant habit of comparing ourselves to others especially during these stressful times.

The Only Valid Comparisons are Those Within Ourselves

How well-prepared are we to face a pandemic, a natural or financial disaster, or another global disruption to our life? Have we done the best we can with what we have? We can only do our best, no more.

> (Coach Kon) *When working with young competitive athletes, I've found that "parents want to compare; players want to compete!" It is not uncommon for parents to draw their own self-worth from the success and level of play of their child. The higher their kid plays, the higher their own status. This artificial comparison creates unnecessary stress and dissatisfaction for the young player, while perpetuating a very*

fragile basis for support by the parent. What happens when the player doesn't make the top team? But he or she is the "best player" on the team! They forget that it is a <u>team</u> sport, and the MVP award goes to the player that makes his or her team mates better because of his or her play. I will never begrudge my players – win or lose – if they have given their best. That's all I can ask of them!

Rather than comparing ourselves to others, we can combine with others to help each other and those less fortunate. Individually we may struggle, but if we pool our resources, if we freely give of ourselves – our resources, our strength, our compassion, our kindness – we will all benefit and overcome the challenges. In a crisis it takes the collective strength and offering of many – each contributing what they have – to get to the other side of adversity. And when we undoubtedly come out on the other side, we will come out stronger as individuals, as families, and as communities.

The Tale of Two Wolves, A Native American Parable

An old Cherokee chief was sitting by the fire and teaching his grandson about life:

> *"A fight is going on inside me,"* he said to the boy. *"It is a terrible fight and it is between two wolves.*
>
> *One is evil. He is anger, envy, sorrow, regret, greed, arrogance, self-pity, guilt, resentment, inferiority, lies, false pride, superiority, self-doubt, and ego.*
>
> *The other is good. He is joy, peace, love, hope, serenity, humility, kindness, benevolence, empathy, generosity, truth, compassion, and faith.*

The same fight is going on inside you and inside every other person too."

The grandson then asked his grandfather, "Which wolf will win?"

The old chief simply replied, "The one you feed."

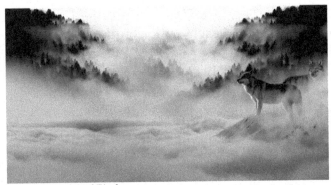

Image from Pexels and Pixabay

Points to Ponder:

- The crucial difference is in how the thought is phrased. If we change the question, we change the path – the direction of our mind is different, and we will therefore come up with different answers.

- All kinds of possibilities will open up, if we give our mind the opportunity to come up with creative solutions, responding to "how" questions, instead of closing the door on ideas by thinking "I can't."

- The feelings and thoughts you focus on will grow inside you and become stronger.

Questions to Consider:

- How does being grateful impact your life?

- Do you compare yourself to others?

Take Action:

Eliminate Negative Thoughts.

- Consider the last time you thought, "I don't have time for _____" or "I can't do _____?" Fill in the blank and rewrite your thought down here:

- Now consider what happens if you change the question to a positive one such as, "How can I find time for _____?" or "How can I make _____ happen?" Fill in the blank space to rephrase the question, and write down the possible answers to the new question here:

Key #7: Kindness

In some ways, the world we live in can make us feel overwhelmed when we contemplate trying to do something to help others. The size of the task alone can make us retreat into our own little world and just try to control that small part of things. But like any endeavor, it requires courage and a first step. Can you help one person? Can you do one thing? We read about tremendous acts of heroism every day, yet most of these people didn't set out to be heroes and save the world. Most of them started with the simple instinct of helping one person in one situation: a kind word of encouragement and compassion in a time of heartbreak, or a plate of food for the hungry. We don't have to perform great or heroic deeds to reap the benefits that come from selflessly giving service to another. **It is the collective efforts of ordinary people doing their part to make the extraordinary possible.**

> *Be kind, for everyone you meet is fighting a hard battle.*
>
> *— Plato*

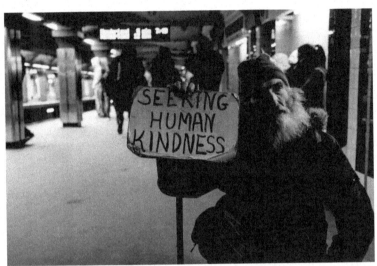

Image by Matt Collamer from Unsplash

Kindness helps both the giver and the receiver

The Greek word for Kindness is *καλοσυνη* (kalosini), meaning the act of a good person wanting to make another happy, wanting well for them. But what impact does kindness have? Can a kind gesture or word give us the hope to keep going, to continue to fight for a better tomorrow? Can it help restore our belief in the goodness of humanity, or help us feel more connected, and less isolated?

We also understand that giving has a positive effect on our own mood and even our overall health. It makes us happy to make a difference in someone else's life! And in her recent book, **The Rabbit Effect**, Columbia University's Dr. Kelli Harding says: *"It helps the immune system, blood pressure, it helps people to live longer and better. It's pretty amazing because there's an ample supply and you can't overdose on it. There's a free supply. It's right there."*

According to author Randy McNeely in his book, **The Kindness Givers' Formula**:

"A natural consequence of both giving and receiving genuine kindness is feelings of gratitude that fill our hearts and the natural lightening of our own burdens and personal challenges. The more we do, the more we experience such amazing feelings of happiness and well-being inside, that we want to do it again, and again, and again.

The Kindness Givers' Formula

4 Simple Steps for Daily Intentional Kindness

DETERMINE	• Determine to be a Kindness Giver
PLAN	• Play ways to be a Kindness Giver
ACT	• Look for and act on opportunities to be a Kindness Giver
INVITE	• Invite and encourage others to be Kindness Givers

Reprinted with permission by Randy McNeely

It's not uncommon for people that have very little themselves, to give generously to others. Perhaps knowing what it feels like to be deprived or in a desperate situation allows them to be more empathetic towards another – even to a stranger. Perhaps it's a need to pay it forward, because they received kindness from someone in the past.

A great example in our lifetime is the work of Mother Theresa, who despite having few possessions of her own, gave freely and completely. As she became more well-known and received support, funds, and world-wide recognition, she never stopped sharing these gifts with those in need. Her kindness changed the lives of so many and served as a glowing example of our higher nature and the transformation that can begin with a single act.

Kind words can be short and easy to speak,

but their echoes are truly endless.

— Mother Theresa

Higher nature, higher angels

It is wonderful, that during a time so filled with negative and fearful events, we are fortunate to see outstanding examples of kindness and compassion, of sacrifice and heroism. We can see our higher angels at work in the brave medical staff and first responders; the people trying to supply our society with the essentials we all need to function; the anonymous voices answering the phone to help others desperately seeking answers to their questions. We have all seen the powerful images from all over the world and closer to home:

- People singing and playing music from their balconies in Italy

- A lone fitness instructor in Madrid, Spain on the roof top helping people quarantined in the surrounding buildings exercise

- Police officers in Marseille, France while patrolling the streets, stopping and engaging entire neighborhoods in a sing-along

- School teachers in the US cruising through their students' neighborhoods, waving and telling them how much they miss them.

Countless examples of the "haves" supporting the "have not's" and the healthy supporting the vulnerable. Celebrities and business leaders pledging money in the hundreds of thousands to hourly workers and support staff unable to work due to the closures. Neighbors grocery shopping for their elderly and high-risk neighbors. So many trying to help as best they can to offer what they have: resources, time, compassion.

When the call went out for healthcare volunteers in New York, 40,000 doctors, nurses, respiratory therapists and other medical professionals signed up within the first days to join a surge health care force to help fight the coronavirus outbreak. More than 6,000 Mental Health Professionals volunteered to offer their services to those suffering emotional and mental distress and trauma during this time.

This phenomenon was repeated across the globe wherever help was needed. Movements were created like the *"Caremongers"* in Canada, and the hundreds of thousand volunteers in the UK and across Europe wanting to help their beleaguered healthcare systems from being overrun by the sheer number of pandemic victims.

When medical staff in communities across the US were desperately low on basic *Personal Protective Equipment (PPE)*, people all over the country pulled out their sewing machines and tools and started producing home-made masks and gowns. Others used their access to 3-D printers to create facemasks and respirator parts.

Chef José Andrés and his non-profit, **World Central Kitchen**, had set up field kitchens to feed thousands of people fresh, nourishing, often hot meals following natural disasters. In the wake of the devastation wrought by Hurricane Maria in 2017, he and his volunteers prepared nearly 4 million meals for residents of Puerto Rico. Considering the global nature of the COVID-19 pandemic, his team quickly moved to distribute meals in low-income neighborhoods in big cities like New York, knowing there would likely be food shortages elsewhere. From small acts of kindness to major commitments, people everywhere have been stepping up to help.

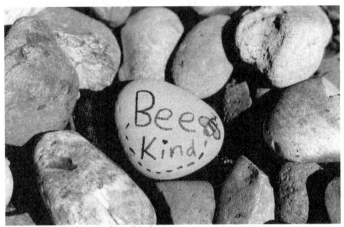

Image by Gerd Altmann from Pixabay

In a world where you can be anything, be kind.

- Unknown

From the Highs to the Lows

Unfortunately, not everyone felt in the giving spirit. It is worth mentioning that there were plenty of individuals and companies trying to profit from others' pain and fear. Hoarding sought-after supplies like hand sanitizer and toilet paper to resell, price-gouging protective equipment like gloves and masks, or encouraging bidding wars for essential life-saving equipment like ventilators. Opportunists sought a quick buck – a "smash and grab" fortune, and they will be remembered for all the wrong reasons.

We also witnessed the willfully ignorant and defiant that disregarded the recommendations of health experts to limit travel and apply social distancing. We witnessed them partying on the beaches during Spring Break and the streets of New Orleans during Mardi Gras, only to contract and spread the Coronavirus and then bring it back to their hometowns like a macabre souvenir. Their sense of entitlement and cavalier attitude hurt not only themselves, but also their families, friends, and other unsuspecting and vulnerable people that would eventually come into contact with them. The label **COVIDIOTS** became popular for those displaying the kind of behavior that purposely ignores health guidelines, jeopardizing one's own safety and the safety of others. But we believe that rather than diminishing the kindness of the many, these poor examples serve to elevate the positive actions even more.

Seek and acknowledge others' reactions

A crisis creates stress for everyone impacted. Anger, fear, anxiety, and frustration can undermine self-confidence and self-esteem, and can ultimately interfere with the success of any attempts to deal with the crisis. At a time of profound dread and uncertainty, we are being cut off from the soothing human contact we so desperately crave. Human touch and physical connection with others – a hug, a handshake, even a high five – are seen as dangerous in the time of the COVID-19 Pandemic!

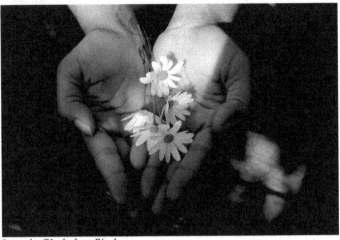

Image by GLady from Pixabay

It is a kindness therefore to encourage others to express their fears, concerns, or needs, and we can help them work through those feelings and refocus on the task at hand. Our empathy can lay the foundation for trust and open communication. Here are some ideas of how we can help:

- Ask other people impacted by the crisis to share their concerns or opinions. Find out what people fear and what they hope will happen. Encourage them to express their frustrations and let them know that their reactions are natural. Share your own concerns, too. Everyone needs to express legitimate concerns about the crisis.

- Be supportive and responsive to people's concerns. Many people who are frustrated by the changes brought on by the crisis frequently lack the information they need in order to adjust and adapt. When a person's job or life change significantly, he or she may not know what to do – or how to do it well. Ask people who are affected by the changes to suggest ideas for overcoming challenges and obstacles. Work with them to develop solutions.

- Be patient. A crisis creates disruption to our routines and forces us to make changes. Even under the best circumstances, people need time to adjust to change. Give them time to work through their emotions and cope with the new reality, even if it's only for the short-term. Try to be accepting of other people's concerns, worries, or behaviors during this time.

Resolve to be tender with the young,
compassionate with the aged
Sympathetic with the striving, and
tolerant with the weak and wrong
Because at some time in your life, you
will have been all of these

— George Washington Carver

When it comes to kindness, everyone wins! So, let's make it a daily habit!

Points to Ponder:

- Kindness is a higher expression of love.

- Kindness brings about change, to both the giver and the recipient.

- Giving to others isn't always convenient . . . but it's always worth it.

Questions to Consider:

- What act of kindness can you perform today?

- How can you make serving others a daily habit?

Take Action:

1. When was the last time you did something out of love?

   (a) What was it? Write it down.

   (b) Do you remember how you felt? Write that down, too.

   (c) How does it feel now, even as you're writing it down? It should bring back the warm feelings.

2. Do something with love for somebody and observe the difference it makes in how you feel when you do it, as well as how you feel afterward. Write down your plan for what you're going to do.

   (a) Write the name of a person for whom you want to do something.

   (b) What are you going to do for them?

   (c) When are you going to do it?

3. Make a commitment to provide service in some way to someone on a monthly basis. Look for an opportunity to serve somebody you wouldn't normally serve.

Write down your plan for the first month:

Conclusion

Beyond a crisis of health, this pandemic has exposed a crisis of trust between people, between individuals and their governments, the experts, the media, and other sources of information. How do we know who to trust? While we look to our experts and our leaders for answers, for direction, we should also listen to are our own intuition, common sense, experience, and inner wisdom. We are empowered to make our own choices, but we are also accountable for the choices we make. After all, **empowerment and accountability are two sides of the same coin**.

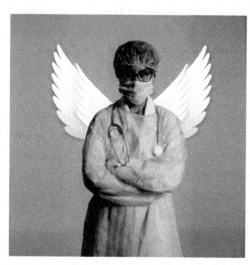

Image by Sathish Kumar Periyasamy from Pixabay

In many ways we are rediscovering the best (and worst) aspects of ourselves. We are rethinking what truly matters most to us and what has value for each of us. When we are placed in situations where we must coexist in confined spaces, aspects of our nature, of our personality – both constructive and destructive – are revealed and on full display.

Reports of domestic violence are growing as people are confined together. People that have been living "parallel lives" together realize they have less in common than they thought, as the isolation and self-quarantining have removed their usual "escapes". These volatile and fragile relationships are impacted further by a very stressful situation, and people struggle to find healthy ways to cope.

On the other end of the spectrum, we see strangers helping strangers. Neighbors that barely exchanged a quick "hello" or a nod of the head in passing each other, are now working to support each other and ensure vital needs are met. Family members and friends we rarely contacted, are now on our screens regularly through the power of video chat applications and technology.

These two extremes illustrate the internal conflicts we all face. To go forward and chase success, or to take the time to be whole and happy. As Arianna Huffington shared in her post, **The Coronavirus is Forcing Us to Ask: What is Truly Essential to Our Life?** In the midst of untold suffering, we are being reminded of something our modern culture has forgotten: that there are two threads running through our lives. One is pulling us into the world to achieve and make things happen, the other is pulling us back from the world to nourish, replenish and refuel ourselves. If we ignore the second thread, it is much harder, especially during these times, to connect with ourselves and with those around us."

It is our ability to come together in these difficult times, to support each other, to encourage each other, that will see us through to better days. What those days will look like, we may not know yet, but we can shape them as individuals and as a community, here and across the globe.

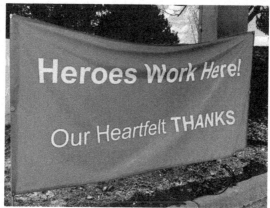

Image by Elia Gourgouris, Ph.D. Avista Adventist Hospital, Louisville, CO

We are Citizens of a Global Community

Every crisis presents an opportunity for exponential change. What do we want tomorrow to look like? What do we want to keep from the "old normal" and use to create our "new normal"? Can we go from surviving this crisis to thriving? This may very well be an opportunity to pivot and take a leap forward as a society of human beings with shared dreams and needs.

Global events require global interventions. No state is immune. No country is immune. These events seldom stop at man-made borders, and easily spill across the lines we draw on the map. A pandemic, a natural disaster, a financial crisis can quickly transcend boundaries.

These are the realities of today's world. Changes to our climate impact all of us. Hot and cold wars leave few of us untouched. The pandemic is impacting all of us directly or indirectly. Soon we will all experience its effects personally in one way or another. We may ourselves fall ill or know someone that has. We may even lose someone close to us.

We need to appeal to our higher nature to do our part, but to also come together, to pool our resources and our knowledge to help each other. This is what helped with previous outbreaks and pandemics – SARS, N1H1, and more recently with Ebola. Humanity is at its best when we all work with transparency and collaboration.

A Final Call to Action

It is our sincere belief that the COVID-19 pandemic is just a warning to humanity and to our way of life. There undoubtedly will be more to come, along with an increasing magnitude and frequency of natural disasters. Global disruptions will also become more common, so we will have to adapt or pay a heavy price, even with our own lives. In the *7 Keys to Navigating a Crisis* we have shared with you both concepts and practical tools to help you deal with these unforeseen events.

It is the ability to choose which makes us human.

- Madeleine L' Engle

It starts with recognizing that we do have a choice as to how we will respond. It may be the only choice we will truly have. Starting with *Self-care*, the ability to put our physical, mental, emotional and spiritual needs first in order to thrive during a crisis.

Practicing *Awareness*, self-reflection and listening to our intuition or inner wisdom will give us advance notice of what's around the corner. Sometimes that can be a matter of life or death.

Choosing *Flexibility* will allow us to adapt, pivot when needed and avoid unnecessary pain. Life will never be the same again and the "new normal" will become the new normal! If we stick to business as usual, we'll be left behind.

The time to act is now, and *Preparation* is key to our survival, then we have succeeded. Preparation is no longer the exclusive domain for a fringe movement of doomsayers but a necessity for all of us.

When faced with a crisis we must take *Initiative* by moving into action. Our response will be determined by the extent of the disaster. Let us not be victims, critics or bystanders. Let us be navigators in the journey of our lives!

As with everything else in life, our *Positive Attitude*, filled with faith and hope will help us overcome any situation and any obstacle we face. More importantly it helps elevate those around us looking for leadership, comfort and a clear vision of getting through the crisis.

Finally, our humanity will be measured by the level and frequency of the *Kindness* we show to others. One of the greatest blessings to come out of the pandemic has been the countless acts of sacrifice, service, and love shown by thousands of ordinary folks doing extraordinary acts of kindness around the world.

Ultimately, will we use this crisis as a way to reset our priorities, or will we go back to the old comfortable way we used to live? If we make the effort and take the time, it's an incredible opportunity to reevaluate our lives, choose what our future priorities will be, and consciously create better lives for ourselves, our families, communities, and our world going forward. Together we can accomplish anything. Humanity demands it of us all and we must rise to the occasion. This is our final call to action!

Be healthy, be safe, and be prepared!

Dr Elia and Coach Kon.

Chapter Notes

Introduction.

1. Arianna Huffington: The Coronavirus Pandemic Is Accelerating Our Mental Health Crisis (https://thriveglobal.com/stories/arianna-huffington-coronavirus-pandemic-accelerating-mental-health-crisis/), thriveglobal.com

2. Depression - World Health Organization (https://www.who.int/news-room/fact-sheets/detail/depression), www.who.int

3. Key Substance Use and Mental Health Indicators in the United States: Results from the 2018 National Survey on Drug Use and Health - Substance Abuse and Mental Health Services Administration (**https://www.samhsa.gov/data/sites/default/files/cbhsq-**), www.samhsa.gov

4. Coronavirus vices like alcohol and eating take a toll on Americans - Axios (**https://www.axios.com/coronavirus-vices-alcohol-marijuana-food-23f02d5e-b82b-4944-8609-b4479af1070e.html**), www.axios.com

5. U.S. online alcohol sales jump 243% during coronavirus pandemic - MarketWatch (**https://www.bloomberg.com/news/articles/2020-04-08/pot-use-reached-all-time-high-in-march-amid-lockdown-measures6.https://www.nytimes.com/2020/04/09/health/coronavirus-smoking-vaping-risks.html7.https://www.marketwatch.com/story/us-alcohol-sales-spike-during-coronavirus-outbreak-2020-04-01**), www.marketwatch.com

6. Pot Use Reached All-Time High in March Amid Lockdown Measures - Bloomberg (**https://www.bloomberg.com/news/articles/2020-04-08/pot-use-reached-all-time-high-in-march-amid-lockdown-measures**), www.bloomberg.com

7. Smokers and Vapers May Be at Greater Risk for Covid-19 - The New York Times (**https://www.nytimes.com/2020/04/09/health/coronavirus-smoking-vaping-risks.html**), www.nytimes.com

8. Coronavirus is changing what we eat: Americans 'craving comfort food' (**https://www.usatoday.com/story/money/2020/04/09/coronavirus-comfort-food-cereal-snacks-baked-goods/2928364001/**), www.usatoday.com

9. COVID-19 Related School Closings and Risk of Weight Gain Among Children - Rundle - - Obesity - Wiley Online Library (**https://onlinelibrary.wiley.com/doi/full/10.1002/oby.22813**), onlinelibrary.wiley.com

10. Personal Health Assessment – By Dr. Elia Gourgouris PhD Copyright 2020

Key 1: Self-Care
1. Lyles, Dr. Terry Stress Recovery- A Disaster Relief Manual, 2005

Key 2: Awareness
1. Bridges, William Managing Transitions: Making the Most of Change, September 22, 2009

Key 3: Flexibility

1. Block Peter, Stewardship: Choosing Service over Self-Interest (San Francisco, Barrett-Koehler Publishers, Inc., 1993, pp. 221-231

2. Siebert, Dr, Al The Resiliency Advantage: Master Change, Thrive Under pressure, and Bounce Back from Setbacks, May 10, 2005

Key 4: Preparedness

1. https://www.ready.gov/

2. FEMA, https://www.fema.gov/

3. Centers for Disease Control and Prevention, https://www.cdc.gov/

4. Pandemic | Ready.gov, **https://www.ready.gov/pandemic**, www.ready.gov

5. Blue Button | HealthIT.gov, (**https://www.healthit.gov/topic/health-it-initiatives/blue-button**), www.healthit.gov

6. https://www.ready.gov/kit

Key 5: Initiative

1. 5, 4, 3, 2, 1: Countdown to make anxiety blast off - Mayo Clinic Health System, (**https://www.mayoclinichealthsystem.org/hometown-health/speaking-of-health/5-4-3-2-1-countdown-to-make-anxiety-blast-off**), www.mayoclinichealthsystem.org

2. Centers for Disease Control and Prevention, (**https://www.cdc.gov/**), www.cdc.gov

Key 6: Positive Attitude

1. Frankl, Victor E. Man's Search for Meaning, June 1, 2006

Key 7: Kindness

1. The Rabbit Effect — Kelli Harding, MD, MPH (**https://www.kellihardingmd.com/the-rabbit-effect**), www.kellihardingmd.com

2. McNeely, Randy The Kindness Givers' Formula, 2019

3. World Central Kitchen (**https://wck.org/?gclid=CjwKCAjwguzzBRBiEiwAgU0FT_3G-baFDjQm-Dm0d41DbkLd8SlTgHvJrcvRETNRP7oFiLS-EzDlMRoCUUsQAvD_BwE**), wck.org

Conclusion:

1. Arianna Huffington: The Coronavirus Is Forcing Us to Ask What Is Truly Essential (**https://thriveglobal.com/stories/arianna-huffington-coronavirus-question-what-is-essential-good-life/?utm_source=Newsletter_AH&utm_medium=Thrive**), thriveglobal.com